The Divine Nature *of* Plants

The
DIVINE NATURE
of PLANTS

A MEDICAL INTUITIVE'S GUIDE TO PLANT SPIRIT MEDICINE

A Sacred Planet Book

Laura Aversano

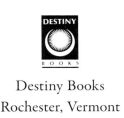

Destiny Books
Rochester, Vermont

Destiny Books
One Park Street
Rochester, Vermont 05767
www.destinybooks.com

Destiny Books is a division of Inner Traditions International

Sacred Planet Books are curated by Richard Grossinger, Inner Traditions editorial board member and cofounder and former publisher of North Atlantic Books. The Sacred Planet collection, published under the umbrella of the Inner Traditions family of imprints, includes works on the themes of consciousness, cosmology, alternative medicine, dreams, climate, permaculture, alchemy, shamanic studies, oracles, astrology, crystals, hyperobjects, locutions, and subtle bodies.

Copyright © 2025 by Laura Aversano

Portions of this book are based upon the author's previous publications of *The Divine Nature of Plants with Wisdom of the Earth Keepers*, published in 2002 by Swan • Raven & Co., and *Plant Spirit Journey: Discover the Healing Energies of the Natural World*, published in 2009 by Llewellyn Publications.

All rights reserved. No part of this book may be reproduced or utilized in any form or by any means, electronic or mechanical, including photocopying, recording, or any information storage and retrieval system, without permission in writing from the publisher. No part of this book may be used or reproduced to train artificial intelligence technologies or systems.

Note to the reader: This book is intended to be an informational guide. The remedies, approaches, and techniques described herein are meant to supplement, and not to be a substitute for, professional medical care or treatment. They should not be used to treat a serious ailment without prior consultation with a qualified health care professional.

Cataloging-in-Publication Data for this title is available from the Library of Congress

ISBN 978-1-64411-445-2 (print)
ISBN 978-1-64411-446-9 (ebook)

Printed and bound in India by Nutech Print Services

10 9 8 7 6 5 4 3 2 1

Text design by Debbie Glogover and layout by Kenleigh Manseau
This book was typeset in Garamond Premier Pro with Orpheus Pro and Mr Eaves Mod OT used as display typefaces

Photos by George M. Sisting

To send correspondence to the author of this book, mail a first-class letter to the author c/o Inner Traditions • Bear & Company, One Park Street, Rochester, VT 05767, and we will forward the communication, or contact the author directly at **LauraAversano.com**.

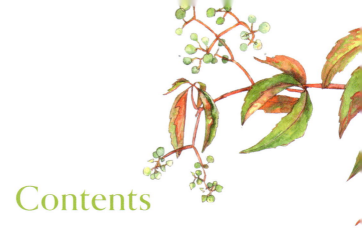

Contents

Foreword by Dr. John Beaulieu — ix

Preface — xi

PART 1
My Journey

1. The Beginning — 2
2. My Shaman — 5
3. Healing Magic — 10
4. Meeting John — 18
5. A Karmic Healing Response — 25
6. Crossing into the Light — 31
7. My Client Work — 42
8. The Appalachians — 58
9. Homecoming — 81

PART 2
Enter into the Divine Nature of Plants

10	The Divine Nature of Plants	98
11	Preparing for the Journey	107
12	The Healing Dimensions and Prayer	112
13	The Plant Spirit Essences	120

PART 3
The Plants, The Spirits, and Their Healing

| 14 | Introducing the Plants | 126 |

Angelica 131

Astragalus 135

Black Cohosh 139

Blessed Thistle 143

Calendula 147

Chamomile 151

Clematis 155

Dandelion 159

Feverfew 163

Lamb's Ear 167

Lavender 171

Lemon Balm 175

Licorice 179

Lilac   183

Marshmallow   187

Motherwort   191

Mugwort   195

Mullein   199

Nettles   203

Poke   207

Pulsatilla   211

Red Clover   215

Rosemary   221

Rue   225

Sage   229

Skullcap   233

St. John's Wort   237

Violet   241

Wormwood   245

Yarrow   249

Guide to the Power of Plants   253

Physical Properties   253

Spiritual and Emotional Properties   260

Index   268

Foreword

Dr. John Beaulieu

It is said that the Buddha once gave a sermon without saying a word; he merely held up a flower to his listeners. I am sure Laura Aversano was in the audience and listening to every word of the Buddha's flower. *The Divine Nature of Plants* is about the art of listening to the spirit essence of each plant. The alchemists called this type of intuitive listening the "law of signatures," and shamans from all Indigenous cultures have learned the art of plant knowledge directly from the plants.

When I read Ms. Aversano's writing, I am reminded of William Blake's poem:

> *To see a world in a grain of sand*
> *and heaven in a wildflower,*
> *hold infinity in the palm of your hand*
> *and eternity in an hour.*

And like William Blake's words, her plant spirit prayers rise to the intensity of poetry to communicate the highest essence of each plant.

In the spirit of Dr. Edward Bach and his discovery of the Bach flower remedies, Laura Aversano honors each aspect of every plant. She listens on many levels and integrates, with ease, her vast intuitive abilities with her knowledge of energy medicine and shamanism. She allows the message of the whole plant to come forward for body, mind, and spirit.

This book is a remarkable work of intuitive listening. Laura Aversano artfully draws us into a world where plants are animated and intelligent beings. Her words are like conduits for the energy of the plants to come to the reader. Something awakens inside of us, and reading and plant healing become one.

Dr. John Beaulieu, ND, Ph.D., is the author of *Music and Sound in the Healing Arts*, *The Polarity Therapy Workbook*, and *The Seven Levels of a Still Point*.

Preface

My communication with souls on the other side, and our united desire to share this marvelous, wisdom-embracing plant spirit medicine with others, is what led me to begin writing this book almost thirty years ago. With the third iteration of this work, my relationship to the earth, its inhabitants, and the enchanted realms imparted to us have increased my respect and awe of the inherent medicine within the natural world. Within these pages you will find the story of my journey, as well as intimate details involving my friends and teachers in the spirit world. You'll read about how I learned to work with plant spirit medicine and how its magic helped both myself and others through difficult times. Following that is a special guide to some of the plants I have worked with over the years to nurture myself, my friends, my family, and my clients. The healing therein will open your heart and mind to a new way of respecting the healing that the natural world has waiting for you. As I have grown over all these years, so have my friendships with the plants and their spirits.

 Because of my energetic sensitivities and openness to high frequencies, my physical body has been plagued by various mysterious ailments since I was a child. Traditional medicine only helped in part. As my relationship with the spirit world grew, I discovered that my life was not my own, in a way, since every experience was leading me closer to my destiny. I eventually came to recognize and align myself with the truth: that I was here to serve, to learn how to heal myself, and to be of assistance to others.

There is a special moment when you realize that there is a distinction between the heavenly world and its spirits, who roam freely, and the earth plane that we physically inhabit. That moment came for me as a child. I was intrigued by spirits, and with psychic abilities that run in my family, I befriended many at a very impressionable age. Some of those spirits later became my allies as I was groomed for what has turned out to be an unimaginable life . . . a life filled with purpose and healing, sorrow and strife, blessing and grace. A life that has embraced many spiritual and physical initiations, starting at the beginning many times over and on many different levels.

Through this book, it is my hope to show how plants and flowers are animate beings that have profound effects on every aspect of humanity and that nature may just be the key to the salvation of humanity.

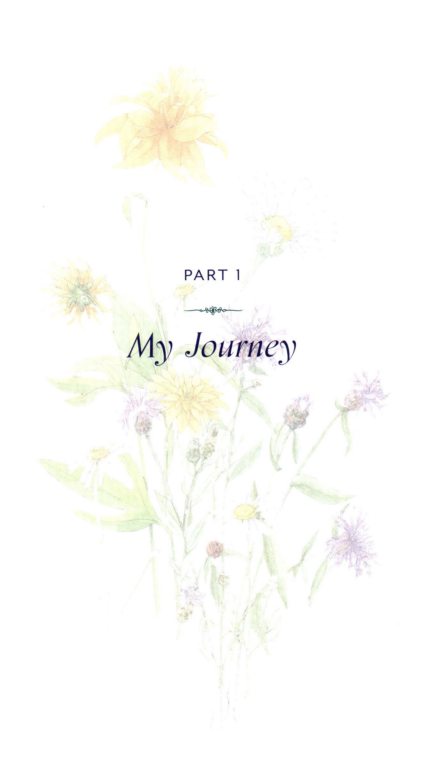

PART 1

My Journey

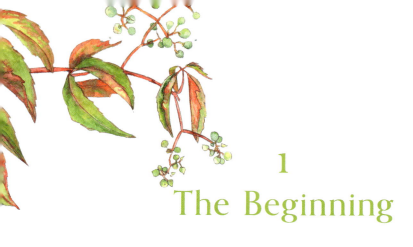

1
The Beginning

When I was a little girl, I would play in the alcove atop my bedroom closet. I often used to think that I was dreaming while awake, since I would see and speak with people that no one else in the house seemed even to notice. I remember telling my mom about my special friends, especially the Native American ones, who would visit and play with me.

By the time I was six or seven, I had developed a keen interest in the afterlife and in souls who could speak and connect with us from beyond the veil. I remembered lives I'd lived before and told my mom how I'd died in some of them. My curiosity about psychic phenomena was beginning to develop, and I am grateful to have had a mother who was gifted as well.

I was plagued with a number of ailments as a child, one of which almost took my life at the age of eight. I had pneumonia and a collapsed lung and was hospitalized for a number of weeks while antibiotics failed to alleviate any of the symptoms that presented themselves. That illness set a precedent for what would be a number of challenging physical conditions throughout my life, conditions that were initiated by the spirit world.

In energy medicine, a "miasm" is an imbalance in the energy field. It can interrupt or corrupt any variable that leads to healing. Miasms can travel with us through various incarnations, and some are passed down in the ancestral DNA of a person's spiritual, emotional, and physical energetic matrix. It is my belief, from years of working with spirits and with clients in my healing practice, that imbalances in the energy field can come from various dimensions and understandings in the spirit world. At the appropriate time and place in a person's life, they will be reconciled.

My miasm was already firmly established by the time I was rushed to the hospital one cold evening in New York City. My heart rate was slow, and I was barely breathing due to the fluid that filled my lungs. I remember being disoriented as nurses and doctors pulled me from the arms of my mother's friend, who was carrying me. Limp and feeling forlorn, I held on to my mother's hand as I drifted into the ethers. I remember the doctors working to find a vein to draw some blood for testing.

I knew that besides my parents, there were other souls around me, ones that no one else could see. And somehow, in the midst of all that chaos, I knew that I would be all right. I had to be. My mother and her father, my grandfather, both had had a spiritual sickness that manifested itself when they were young. As was the case with me, the traditional route to healing was of little avail for them.

As my mother remembers the story from her native Sicily, my grandfather fell ill at a very young age. His symptoms mimicked a coma in today's pathology, but back then all the local doctor knew was that there was a young boy who would not wake up. After every method of waking my grandfather failed, a decision was made to call the witch doctor who lived on that part of the island. After many prayers, and with my grandfather still in a coma, the witch doctor summoned my grandfather to get up and get one of the family's chickens, cut off its head, and then to come back to the bed.

That's all my mother can recall of the story. Obviously, my grandfather eventually awakened from his comatose state. No one could have foretold that he would have a special child later in his life—my mother, who was never able to come to the fullest realization of her gifts, even to this day.

The spiritual pattern that afflicted my grandfather was passed on to my mother, and eventually to me. I don't know all the genealogical history in my family, but I'm sure this spiritual pattern began before my grandfather was born.

When my mother was a young girl, she too went into a coma-like state and was actually being prepared for burial rituals when she awoke. She apparently had been "dead" for a number of hours. The local doctor could not get a heartbeat from her, and no one knew what had occurred. She says that when she awoke she was surrounded by faces staring at her, initially in horror at her resurrection. Then there was joy. Later on, they theorized that she might have had some sort of anaphylactic reaction to shellfish she'd consumed. But my mom has continued to gorge on shellfish all her life, without the slightest hesitation or consequence. She is indeed special, a chosen one of the gods and spirits. She still says that she thought she was dreaming every time the Holy Mother appeared at the foot of her bed, yet she traversed the streets of her town praying litanies to her. She never knew how she came to know the words of those prayers, but people would follow her and join in.

In my case, after a number of days in the intensive care unit, I was transferred to a regular bed at New York Hospital. There, I recovered slowly—the prescribed antibiotics still a futile strategy as far as I was concerned. When I left the hospital, I knew I was different. I couldn't explain it then, as an eight-year-old, but I can explain it as I look back now. It is simple: I was no longer a child of this world only. I had been initiated into what would become an intense, intriguing, beguiling, and very challenging spiritual path for years to come.

The miasm had been passed to me not as a burden, but as an opportunity to heal the ancestral imbalances, if you will, of the generations before me. I guess God knew what he was doing, but I could never have imagined the life I was about to live.

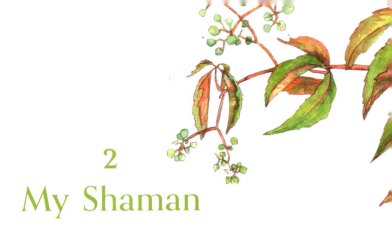

2
My Shaman

Years later, the fragmented pieces of my spiritual path began to make sense . . . especially after I befriended a 2,000-year-old shaman in the spirit world who would later come to guide and protect me.

One day when I was in my late twenties, I was walking the streets of New York, my physical body visible to the naked eye but my spirit lurking between the worlds. I was praying for someone to help me in the midst of my healing crisis. With my shoulders hunched against the rain-drenched air, I walked slowly, asking the spirits for a healer, for a magician imbued with the teachings of white magic. I needed an herbalist, a dreamer, a spirit walker. Carrying my medicine bag and gifts for the one I knew must appear, I meandered impatiently and hopefully, trusting that the spirits would soon send someone to assist me.

Despite my years of training in the healing arts, my studies in various spiritual traditions, my training in shamanic work, and my abilities as a medium, I had nothing but my faith to go on in asking for this help. The miasm was beginning to heal on a different level, and I needed a way to move beyond it.

I was shielding my face from a cool drizzle that felt more like ice crystals when I heard small footsteps behind me. I knew they were coming from the spirit world. I stopped, held my breath, and waited to hear the footsteps again. There was silence. I waited another moment before

I began to walk again . . . and there they were: tiny, mysterious, yet effulgent footsteps. Then a bright light began to emanate as an indomitable soul came forth: a shaman.

He looked at me quizzically, and through telepathic means let me know that he followed the traditions of his grandfathers. That meant that speaking to women was somehow inappropriate, but because of all the work I had done on behalf of the spirit world in the past, he deemed my "call" worthy enough to be answered. (As a medium, I expect spirits simply to talk to me or give me visions—this was the first time a spirit used telepathy to relay his intentions.) He let me know that he was fully aware of why I was there; I didn't need to repeat myself. I was so in awe of his impeccable demeanor, and of a discipline I knew I could never harness, that I was trying not to laugh. He continued our "conversation" telepathically, letting me know that he would help and showing me how things were beginning to come full circle. Our conversation seemed to last for hours, yet in this earthly reality it was only minutes. He knew of my work as a medium and healer and was seemingly pleased about my work with plant medicine. After all, he was trained as a shaman in the ritual use of plant spirit medicine. As a spirit walker, he continues to utilize these gifts, imparting them to those of us in this earthly reality and also to his fellow brethren in the ethers. As we talked, he was accessing my memories on a soul level, letting me know through clairvoyant and clairsentient means what he was seeing . . . pictures of my childhood, of my initiations, of all the souls who stayed near me from beyond, and of the many remedies that had been given to me over the years to help me heal myself and those who came to me. The plethora of remedies and natural healing cures I had always used in my work came from souls like this shaman. I like to think of these souls as the plant gods.

The plant gods are the teachers and medicine healers of the plants. They have numerous responsibilities. They can summon plant spirits, or plant elementals (fairies, elves, devas, gnomes, and other spirits of nature) at will. They perform plant magic, encourage the relationship between humans and elementals, and facilitate great depths of spiritual healing within and between the worlds. The plant gods are travelers and exist anywhere in the time and space continuum where souls reside. They are granted certain privileges to heal karma and to work with negativity. They act as a conduit between altered states of reality—this is what enables humans to work with the elementals surrounding the plants. My shaman is himself a plant god, and he came to help me. To this day he has never given me his name, and he still does not communicate with me verbally, only through telepathic means.

As far as plant elementals go, the main thing to remember is that a different elemental will come to each person who works with prayer and plant magic. And a different elemental will come to each plant god who invokes it. Each elemental will have a different teaching on how to best utilize the healing properties of the plant medicine, and the way in which one elemental connects with the plant will be different from how another connects. Likewise, how a human being receives, interprets, and utilizes plant magic will vary from person to person. The manner in which a plant god allocates higher meaning and the vibrational connection between a human and an elemental is up to that plant god.

That cold rainy day was the first time I stood in the presence of my shaman, that sentient being, as he held me in his magic. My body was somewhat erect as I felt his "words" penetrate me. My spirit, weak and sullen, was somehow made stronger by the energies this plant god imparted. The dreamlike state I was in was surreal, even more so because I was utterly exhausted from the spiritual work I had been doing lately. The city block where I encountered the shaman was lined with magnificent pine trees, and I could feel him invoking the trees as he worked with me, calling upon the elementals that he felt could bring me healing. They listened, and they came without hesitation. It was as though the leaves and branches positioned themselves in my direction to protect me, and you could hear the sound of soft whistling in the wind. The air had an etheric feeling and a sense of light pulsation to it, something I am familiar with and attribute to the presence of spirits hovering. He called upon them, one and all, to breathe magic into me and give me hope. It was his prayer, undeniably and exuberantly so.

The shaman's prayer was unspoken, and its vibration traversed every state of consciousness, both tangible and intangible to human senses. Its power was illuminated by the purity of the shaman's intention. And it all happened so fast, as I was passing in and out of some kind of altered state. Something else was unfolding here—a higher level of communication, another level of consciousness and healing.

There is no time boundary when among the spirits, and the hours that passed in my mind lasted only a few minutes in reality. I was in a stupor when the elementals departed. The shaman, as indomitable as ever, left quietly and walked off into the ethers. He didn't even say goodbye. The gift I had prepared, of stones, hair, and flowers, was now for him, and I sang a song as I looked for a place to lay these intricacies down. I found a home for my offering by one of the trees and didn't even notice the myriad of people walking to and fro, passing me without observing my bewilderment.

I went home and rested. My meeting with the shaman had been extraordinary. Over the next few months, he returned to show me how my work with the spirit world, specifically with the plant gods, was to release me from the miasm, from the pattern I was born into. This work with plants would also assist me in my efforts to help souls on the other side who are bound to this earth by their own struggles; I would be able to ask the plant spirits for intercession on behalf of souls, and would learn more about the vibrational healing capacities that each living plant embodies, and how that vibration can mirror a thought, emotion, or illness in the earth realm.

But while is easy for me to call upon spirit guides or other souls in the ethers, such is not the case with my shaman. He is a busy soul and respects the hierarchy of grandfather healers from which he descends.

In recent years he has not visited as often as he did during that turbulent and inspiring time when I first met him, but I know where to find him if I have need of him.

In my many years working with clients before I met the shaman, I had received remedies from various healing spirits. These remedies embraced every aspect of human nature and originated in the plant, mineral, and animal kingdoms. I'd always had a relationship with the spirits who imparted the knowledge. But rarely did I have a relationship with the remedies themselves—and that is what my shaman came to teach me. He wanted me to develop a more personal relationship with the remedies, especially those that came from plants. Meeting the shaman seemed to open a new dimension of the spirit world to me; I now had access to the spirits within this dimension, their healing powers, more remedies than I'd known before, and many new truths about working with plant elementals and spirits of that nature. My awareness was greatly increased, as was my potential to work on another level. For this I am profoundly grateful.

My shaman let me know that, in order to build a more personal relationship with the plant remedies, I needed to be initiated into another dimension of the spirit world and go through a series of healing crises and upheavals. Only after those experiences could I convey my new knowledge. My shaman wanted the new knowledge to heal me and also wanted me to draw on it to heal others.

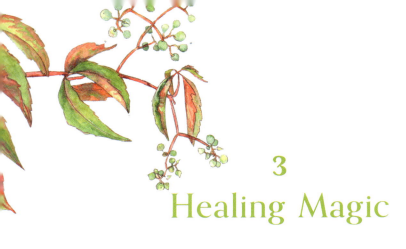

3
Healing Magic

I had begun to experience various healing crises and upheavals before I ever met my shaman, which is why I was walking the streets of New York, searching for a soul who could help me. Physically, I was having a severe allergic reaction to pesticides that were being sprayed in my area for mosquitoes, and spiritually, I had been working with the souls of some lost children who were somehow stuck in the ethers, more or less earthbound and not knowing how to be released into the light.

Every summer, for several years, spray trucks had ventured into my neighborhood to kill mosquito larvae. The pesticides were sprayed with little concern for human health and well-being or for the environmental devastation they caused, and with little or no advance warning. The first year that the government sprayed, a strong neurotoxin was used that affected many people. My immune system couldn't take the harsh chemicals that seeped through my nervous system, and I was sick for months. The second year, they changed the pesticide, but it still left me debilitated and working hard to clear my body of the harmful residue. By the third year, I thought that I might have built up a resistance to it, but I hadn't. A month after they sprayed, I developed seizure-type episodes. I spent months trying to repattern my nervous and immune systems and hours receiving acupuncture treatments and cranial-sacral work. My nutrition focused on increasing essential fatty acids in my diet and any other brain foods I could think of. I also worked with herbs and homeopathy to cleanse out my liver.

Throughout this time, I knew that my work with the lost children in the spirit world also had something to do with my physical condition. I knew that my prayers had to be strong, both for myself and for those whom I was asked to help. Although I had some sort of plan, holistically speaking, it still felt like I was chasing my tail. Something was missing—so I sat down one day and came up with a new strategy. I needed to invoke the spirit world as only I knew how and ask what they needed from me to help me move beyond my malady. I also wanted them to teach me how to work with the toxins in my body on a different level.

> Crazy Horse dreamed and went into the world where there is nothing but the spirits of all things. That is the real world that is behind this one, and everything we see here is something like a shadow from that world.
> — Black Elk

A major part of this new plan was meeting a spirit who would come and assist me. I knew I would have to go through a metamorphosis, and I balked at the idea of having to endure some of the trials I knew would come, but I had no choice. I was stuck. My body wasn't able to rebalance and rid itself of the pesticide residue, and the lost children were constantly around me, sometimes playing, sometimes crying, attaching themselves to me to such a degree that other clairvoyant mediums could see them around me. Their energies were very heavy, since they were frightened and their souls were very old. I was stuck, they were stuck, and we were going nowhere together.

After I met my shaman, I could always tell when he was present, since the vibration and energy in the air around me would shift. The light would deepen, and the walls would look like shadows in a multidimensional structure that enclosed me. I always waited patiently for his visits, and little by little, he imparted instruction and healing—my initiation into the work with plants had begun. I was addled by his methodology, but it didn't matter; I needed his help and took down some notes. I was still bewildered as to how the lost children could help my physical body convalesce and how the plant magic would play into all of this.

To explain my relationship with the lost children, I should first share some of my own spiritual practices. When I pray in the morning, I always pray for the souls in purgatory and in other dimensions of the spirit world. I was raised Catholic and revere the teachings of the Christian saints and martyrs, especially when it comes to the repose of a soul. I also embrace the Buddhist teachings of reincarnation and have somehow intertwined the two so that they fit my understanding and development. Many times during prayer and in my state of contemplation, souls come and go around me, asking me to pray for them. Simple enough. As a Catholic, I draw from the many wonderful prayers that have been passed down through the ages, especially prayers for souls who are not at rest. I also devote time to creating my own sacred words for the heavens.

One memorable day, I was saying a prayer to St. Joseph to benefit children, specifically the ones who had been coming to me. One by one, they entered the living room where I sat silently and began to laugh and move in concentric circles around me. They made me laugh, and I tried not to pay too much attention to them as they watched me. I wasn't sure why I was even praying for them, since they seemed so happy. New children always came each day, and some of the ones who had visited me previously would return. I usually would laugh with them for a moment, then return to my novenas.

But on this day, my curiosity got the better of me and I sat with them for a while, wondering where they had come from and why they were there. One of them took me through the spirit world to an orphanage in Europe during the late 1800s or early 1900s and showed me that some of the children who had been visiting me had died there of the plague. The care they received was dismal, and most of them longed for companionship. Their clothes were thin and tattered, their stomachs distended from starvation, and their teeth rotting from malnutrition. They came to me "happy" because they lived each day in the orphanage in a state of make-believe. They pretended to be joyful and carefree, with warm meals filling their tummies and shoes with laces that were as strong as steel, ones that wouldn't break during their free-spirited play. They played both by themselves and with one another, but often were sickly. They mostly stayed inside the orphanage, looking through the dirt-stained windows to get a glimpse of the outside world.

There were other children who visited me as well, from various places and times in earthly reality. The common thread seemed to be that they had all been abandoned in some manner. Some had been abused, many had lived on the streets, and many died from disease. All in all, I got to "meet" them and hear their stories.

But how were these children connected to my physical condition, and how was the shaman going to help me? How was I going to learn what he wanted me to learn about his work with plant medicine? It all seemed overwhelming to me, but as the children kept coming and staying near, my body would feel their illnesses, and their emotions would run through me. There were days I was stronger and days I was weaker. I continued to do the same self-care things I'd always done, while awaiting the next steps from my new spirit friend.

The shaman came every so often at the beginning, bringing me healing energy. He would use his prayers and plant magic. The first time he asked me to lie down on my living room floor, so that he could do some healing work on me, was memorable. As he came near, other souls began to come out of the ethers and gather with him around me. He called upon them, and then, with his prayers, he called upon the plants. He summoned one plant in particular: *Phytolacca americana*. Poke.

The spirits and souls around me were preparing the plant for me. It is a miraculous thing to behold spirits bringing you healing. Although I wasn't able to see the plant elementals who were present, I could perceive them through clairaudience and clairsentience; the spirits and souls around me all seemed to be aware of the elementals springing forth. Their relationship with the elementals was one of beneficence and complete trust. I then understood that these spirits and souls were plant gods. And the elementals—the spirits of many different plants—were their joyful cohorts.

The shaman wanted to show me one of the lifetimes where this miasm of mine began. I was one of them, a medicine woman in the Native American tradition. I was suffering from what looked like a bout of tuberculosis. A healer was making an herbal preparation for me, and I went through a cathartic healing crisis before I became well. It looked like they'd called upon the poke plant back then, as well. There were children around me in that lifetime, playing. Some of them had stayed with me; their lightheartedness was what had attracted some of the lost children who also were now at my side. Apparently I'd never let them go. Then the vision of myself in that lifetime dissipated, and I continued to stay present with the healing that the spirits were facilitating for me.

The spiritual energies of the poke plant were like an aphrodisiac. The spirits seemed to dance around me with the preparation that they made, and their laughter was so voluminous that I couldn't contain myself and joined in. I could tell that they were releasing some kind of held energy within me, physically, emotionally, and spiritually. My laughter turned into coughing and a metallic taste formed on the tip of my tongue. I knew that I was ridding some of that pesticide residue from my system. My coughing went deeper, until I was able to push up some mucus, and then it subsided. There was an emptiness within and around me. Something had given way in my chest, and all I could feel was the emptiness.

My past life as a medicine woman no longer seemed to hold any energy in my energy field, and I knew that some of the lost children had made their way into the light. It was only a handful, but it was a start. I felt empty, even sad, and I realized how tightly I was holding on to souls that I didn't even know were attaching to me so strongly. I'd probably been doing this since the day I was born. I wondered whether, if my thinking had not been so myopic, I could have helped these children into the light any earlier, through prayer.

I guess it didn't matter. The timing was right, and perhaps there was more meaning than I realized in their attachment to me. As I lifted myself up, the shaman was still around me, but the other souls had vanished. The etheric mist that accompanies the spirit world was very profuse. I could breathe better—I could definitely feel that—and something had shifted for me physically. Later, when I looked at myself in the mirror, I saw that my coloring was not as yellow as it had been since the spraying of the pesticides began. I had many questions, but the shaman wasn't about to give me many answers. This was going to be a memorable relationship and apprenticeship.

When those few lost children crossed into the light, they had taken some of the poison out of my body so that I could really begin to heal. And some of the internal inflammation that I had tried to calm through other means had shifted slightly. Even my eyesight was a little better, for a while. I knew that there had to be reasons why the children had been with me for all those years, but it didn't really matter. Now just seemed to be the time to start healing this miasm. The teacher had appeared, and the work had begun. I did want to know more about the poke plant that day, since it was obviously very strengthening for me. When I asked the shaman about it, he prayed, as though getting permission from a higher source to impart the knowledge. He then began to show me some of its healing properties. He didn't call upon the elementals again to dictate the plant magic; rather, he simply funneled it in a way that I could see it for myself. He was trying to teach me not just about connecting to the plant elementals, but also about connecting with the gods who have dominion over them.

When the shaman invoked poke, his lips formed subtle syllables as he raised his head toward the sky. I could hear only what appeared to be mumbling . . . perhaps a song, a prayer. He sang what came to him; he sang what came through him. I felt the energy come down through my crown chakra, into my heart, and ground through the earth. His prayer was as melodious a chant as I have ever heard. Even though its words would seem inane, if even audible, to a normal person, they made sense to me because of their vibration.

He let me see for a brief moment into the window of his world, of his spiritual makeup, of his gifting from the One Creator. And I saw poke through his eyes. Tears started to roll down my cheeks as my own prayer began to form, words like butterflies flying effortlessly from my lips to God's ears:

Great Creator and Spirit of the Buffalo, we surrender to your powerful medicine. We stand here before you, seeking guidance and direction. Bring to us your wisdom, Great Spirit, so that we may follow in the trails you leave behind. Show us the way, for we are your children.

I was hearing the words in my head, and the melody was ringing in my voice. Wow—that was my prayer. When my spirit reached out to the soul of the poke plant, the prayer just began to emanate from my lips. The joy I felt in this sacred communion was illuminating. The emptiness I'd felt just a few moments before, after the healing, was now filled. My heart and soul felt whole. I had released something back to spirit—some of the children—and it felt like this connection, this joy, was their gift to me in return.

The soul is an empty vessel, but the Creator looks at emptiness much differently than we do. There is great splendor in finding union, and great ecstasy in creating a relationship with the Higher Power. All things stem from the Creator, and all unions are meant to be made in the image and likeness of our union with the Creator. There is emptiness as we search aimlessly for this connection, and there is utter bliss when we find it.

> From an aboriginal point of view, no one can accomplish anything who is not in alignment with the gods or a God.
> *Malidoma Some*

In my prayer to poke, I had found that bliss for a moment. I looked at my shaman, and gratitude filled my heart for his kindness toward me. Before he left the room, he helped me to see some of poke's healing qualities. Later, I would learn more about this plant from the elemental that came to me. At the moment, however, I was receiving transmissions of energy directly from the plant god—my shaman—and knowledge about poke directly from him. Here are some of the images and wisdom I received for poke:

This amazing creation of nature can bring warmth and love to one's heart. It can alleviate fear and anxiety and help promote a deep sense of faith and trust in self and in one's spiritual path. Poke heals broken spirits throughout all creation. It is a plant of enormous strength and is used for protection. It can induce trancelike states of consciousness for purposes of healing.

There was more; there was much more. I knew these healing messages were meant for me, but I felt that others would benefit from them as well.

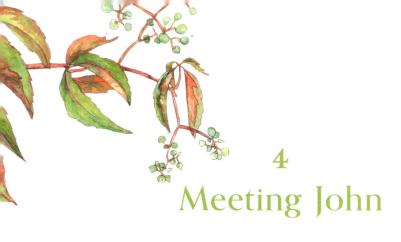

4
Meeting John

After the shaman left, I knew I had some work to do. One of the first instructions he'd given me, during our previous conversations, was about helping a male soul who was unable to cross into the light. Since I was receiving help myself, it was my obligation to help others. I had listened to the shaman, not really knowing the direction I was headed and not sure what he had in mind. But I had faith in him.

When he asked me to visit the local cemetery, I thought he was crazy. I don't especially like cemeteries, since earthbound souls sometimes linger there. But the next day I got in my car and drove for about five minutes. The cemetery is one of the largest in this part of New York City, and I didn't have a clue where to go. I prayed and then was guided to drive down a narrow street and park my car near the cemetery gates that were open. I figured that the shaman would meet me there.

I got out of my car and hesitantly walked through the aisles of gravestones. I took with me my rosary, a candle, my prayer books, and some gifts of flowers. I looked around to make sure the caretaker or another employee of the cemetery was nowhere near—I was afraid if they saw me with all those trinkets, I would get kicked out. As I was walking, I called upon the shaman and asked him to show me where I was supposed to go. I glanced at the hundreds of headstones until my eyes came upon what looked like a portal of light. Below the portal was a small and very antiquated headstone, next to a glorious tree. I looked around, just to make sure I wasn't seeing things or that the light wasn't above any other headstone.

I waited a few moments, then walked over to the grave site and laid my tools on the ground. I sat under the tree. It was autumn and the ground was a little cold and bare. I felt uneasy and began to question everything. Did I really need to go this route? I was very glad that the shaman had come into my life, but was the path I was taking going to bring me healing? More importantly, would peace come to those lost children who had embedded themselves in my energy field and, ultimately, in my home? I wasn't sure. And I was tired. I wanted to bargain—I was willing to do the work that was needed to fully heal, but I didn't want to add any more to my plate if it wasn't necessary. I went back and forth with these thoughts for a few minutes, wondering again whether, if I stayed true to my holistic modalities, within time the pesticides would fully clear from my immune and nervous systems. And I wondered if, with unceasing prayer, the lost children would finally come to rest.

I was jolted out of my indecisive musings by a grounds keeper who asked if I was okay. I told him yes and thanked him for checking up on me. He didn't say anything about the spiritual tools that were on the ground in front of me. I guess he just assumed that I was praying for someone that I'd lost. He went away, and I gave my attention to the headstone surrounded by light. I don't remember the exact inscription. I do, however, remember that the name was John and that he died in the early 1900s. There wasn't anything remarkable about his headstone; it was actually pretty ordinary and felt lonesome to me. I wondered who John was and why I was there to help him.

So how do you call upon a soul in the spirit world? I just ask for them. And I tell my clients the same thing—just call spirits by name. Either they will come or, if your prayers are fervent, someone else who can give you messages about them will come. So I called. I called John.

My face began to glow with warmth, which usually happens when I open up to the spirit world. I called John, and alternately, I called my plant god, my shaman.

"John, my name is Laura. I'm not sure what I am doing here, but I'm supposed to pray for you. I don't know if you can hear me or even want to hear me; I just want you to know I'm here. I don't mean to bother you, but you feel kind of lonely to me, and I was wondering if there was anything I could do for you." I didn't hear anything. I didn't know if I would hear him, or see him, or both. I took my red-beaded rosebud rosary and began praying the Divine Chaplet, and with that, the Catholic prayers for eternal rest. As I repeated the same prayer with each delicate rosebud bead, the portal seemed to grow bigger and bigger, and the light seemed to emanate in all directions.

I kept going until I began to notice that an energy was present. I was enervated by it. My heart began to pound and become weak, and I became aware that there was some anger and bitterness present. I knew that the presence wasn't my shaman, so it had to be John.

"John, is that you?" I asked. I didn't hear a response, but my body was mirroring his more and more, so I knew I had to hold a stronger boundary. I could also tell that John had been a smoker when he was alive. I repeated myself. "John, are you there?" Still, no one answered. I could tell he was frightened; I could tell he was lost. I could feel that he didn't trust anybody. Sometimes this happens with a spirit when a medium is trying to make a connection. The soul may not want to speak up, or it may take a while for them to trust you, especially if they have been wandering the earth as a lost soul for years. When this happens, it has been my experience that other souls who are very aware of this soul will intercede on their behalf and do the communicating.

I felt it was him, and that he was observing my every move from beyond the veil. I called to my shaman for help, and to any other spirits who could give me a little more insight into John's earthbound reality. And boy, did they come. A number of John's family members who had not been able to reach him before came. They had been looking for him, but for some reason could not find him. They had been waiting a long time to be reunited with him. Through these spirits, I got to see a little of John's life. He seemed to be a midshipman, a sailor, I think for the navy. He lost the love of his life early on and stayed alone for the rest of his years. He didn't really spend much time associating or socializing with others, but mostly kept to himself. He seemed to be a handsome man—tall, with light eyes and hair strewn across his head. This information was not coming to me from John but from those who loved him most, as well as from my spirit guides. John's gravestone looked untouched and inviolable, as though it had not been visited or disturbed in years.

Melancholy came over me as I tried to reach out to John directly, but it was of no avail. I kept praying and turned my vision to the shaman. I asked him to intercede and help John, or at the very least show me how to help him. The shaman asked me to be patient with John. While the methods I am accustomed to were helping, they didn't seem to be enough, which is why I thought my plant god might have another way.

There is always more than one way to help a soul who is stuck. There are many spiritual traditions that offer rites of passage and ceremonial tributes to the dearly departed. There are also thousands of prayers devoted to the dead. My shaman's way of helping souls is simply one of these many approaches—one that I was going to learn.

I looked at my shaman intently. My eyes were dazzled by the gleaming sunlight that seemed to land right in front of my feet, near the headstone. I waited, and he watched. Then he took his staff and lifted it up to the sky, as though embracing the omnipotence of the spirits of nature. In my psychic vision, his brown skin radiated with gentleness and such utter faith that the sight left me motionless. I don't even remember taking a breath. He began to mumble, like he had done before; unrecognizable syllables emanated from his lips. He was one with his words, and his eyes were lowered in reverence, even though his head was tilted toward the sunlight.

He was saying his prayer, invoking the plant spirits. I wasn't privileged to see which of the elementals he was invoking; my attention was focused on the sweet melody that reverberated with each breath he took. It went on and on, and it was glorious. I glanced at the tree above me, and I could swear that the leaves were dancing to his prayer. They were smiling to his song. There were still some green leaves left, even though autumn hues graced the entirety of the tree. And they were luminous—every red, auburn, burnt-orange, green, pointed, withered leaf. Luminous, every one of them. And they knew they were being summoned.

When a plant spirit is summoned, all of nature listens, and many elementals will answer the call, even if just for support. So when one is called, all embark. The responsibility may be left to only one elemental, or it can be left to many; that is the decision of the plant god. Thus, the trees glistened, the sun shone even brighter, the clouds above formed what looked like celestial shapes, and the birds came nearer to where I sat. Others could only see a woman, with her rosary and some religious oddities, sitting on the ground by a headstone. But to me, I was in the presence of greatness—a sea of spiritual beings and souls who wanted to serve. I was in awe.

Even the headstones in the cemetery seemed to awaken—or rather, the souls attached to them awakened. I felt blissful. The souls around John started to pay attention to the song, and eventually, so did John. They didn't see the shaman; they did see me, though. And they responded to his prayer to the plant spirits. They clasped their hands in the hopes that this prayer would reach John in some way. I saw John looking for the source of this heavenly inspiration. I could feel him look my way to see if I was singing this prayer, and I obviously could not take the credit. When I saw that he was responding, I continued praying with my rosary so that John could receive all the help that he needed.

His energy started to brighten as his curiosity grew. Where was this sacred sound coming from? The vibrations were so strong that it seemed to open a portal so that John could see the family members who were waiting for him. He looked at them. His shoulders loosened, as did his protective stance. His chest muscles seemed to relax in a way that they hadn't in lifetimes. He looked up and gazed at what I believe was light. The gloominess and shadowing that had marked his facial features seemed to lift.

My heart lightened, as though my own burdens were dissipating. It was as if I were in the midst of a family reunion that was hundreds of years overdue. John's demeanor changed dramatically, and the overtones in the air seemed to quell any anxieties that John had about my disturbing him. My shaman continued to sing his prayer, and tears welled up in my eyes. I had totally forgotten that I was sitting in the middle of New York City, in one of the largest cemeteries in the county, on an autumn day, under a tree, in a front of a headstone of a man I had never known.

The air started to clear, and as quickly as John and his relatives came, they made their way together into the next dimension—the light that was awaiting them. My shaman stayed, and the other helping spirits who supported us departed. It is not uncommon for me to feel a great emptiness when I come out of such a high vibration of souls and spirits, to rest gently in the arms of earthly reality. That emptiness was present now, even though one soul was left, and he was still praying.

I asked the shaman if it was appropriate for him to tell me which plant elemental he'd called upon, specifically, to help John in his crisis. Like last time, I waited. And then I started to hum. It felt like my heartstrings were being tickled, and I hummed even louder. Then from my lips, a prayer to lemon balm came, and with it, the elemental—who wanted to show herself to me.

Fly, little fairy, as fast as you can, and bring magic to each lemon balm with the stroke of your hand. Using your wand, filled with God's grace, make nectar of its leaves for the entire human race.

I repeated the prayer as quickly as it came, over and over again, my head spinning with dizziness at the burst of energy that accompanied the prayer. As I spoke, a little effervescent fairy came whizzing by. She was delicate but strong, and in her tiny hand she carried a wand of magic. She alighted upon each leaf of the lemon balm plant in the spirit world and tapped her wand to activate the healing magic of the plant.

She told me she would come to me again at a later time to share more of her magic and how she imparts it to help humans, but she wanted to share with me now some of the healing qualities that her magic brings to people.

She let me know that lemon balm is the plant of gathering for spiritual communion. My shaman had called upon her and, by virtue of his power, was able to intensify and bridge the karmic connections that exist between the plant kingdom and the human world. She heeded my shaman's call and came into the energy sphere with John and his family members and helped to open the portal that healed the rift. The fairy helped John overcome his fear of being in the world, both the one he'd lived his last existence in and the dimension he resided in now. She brought him courage and helped to soothe his soul and the grief he'd carried for years. She brought immediate comfort to his heartache and helped put his wandering mind at ease.

With his heart healed, he was able to be free.

I was tired. I left the cemetery, feeling much more peaceful than when I'd arrived, and went home.

5
A Karmic Healing Response

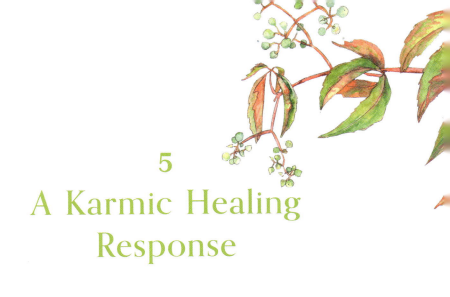

Over the next few days, I went into yet another healing crisis. My skin turned a pale yellowish color, my hair became brittle again, and my skin seemed tauter. I went to bed each night with my body burning as though I had been through a chemical reaction. I was sweating, and my face would swell. My body would shake as if I had the chills, but internally, I always felt feverish. I would lie there in bed until some of the symptoms subsided. It was always the worst at nighttime.

During the day, I was mindful of my diet and the supplements I was taking. I would eat, lightly, foods that would continue to cleanse my liver and gallbladder. I spent time doing castor oil packs and taking salt-and-baking-soda baths. Herbal plant baths were also part of my agenda. Whatever I needed to do to get through this healing crisis, I would do it. In response to my prayers, the spirits assured me that I was just detoxing from the poisons in my body. They even let me know beforehand what would occur, to lessen any fear that I might have. I have always trusted in these helping spirits, who relay healing information to me. They have dictated information that I have shared with my clients over the years.

During this time, I often looked at an angel statue my sister had given me one Christmas, and whenever I psychically saw her face swell up or her eyes get red, I knew that this would happen to me as well. It is commonplace for objects belonging to a person to take on their energy, which is why psychics can look at someone's picture or hold a piece of clothing and tell a lot about a person. My home and the things in it have taken on my energy, so it is easy for me to see what might be going on within myself if I look at my possessions. And it wasn't just the angel statue that confirmed what was happening to me—all the statuary in my home told me things about my health. I used these psychic visions as confirmation of what I heard from the spirits in my prayers.

Also, during such healing crises, I found myself under spiritual duress, torment, and attack. I was more open and vulnerable because my body was so weak and my boundaries were permeable. I spent a lot of time at my local chapel whenever this occurred, and much time doing protection rituals. I needed to pray often, and spiritual cleansing became my ordinary reality. When I was this sensitive, I would stay clear of large groups of people or busy places, anything that held frenetic energy. I just knew it wouldn't be good to put myself in a position of taking on more energy. I would also distance myself from people or places that held a lot of negative energy and those places where a lot of souls tended to gather and wander. It is part of the work, and part of what I need to do to respect the nature of who I am and the gifts that were given to me.

During those healing crises, I was lucky to have support from friends, colleagues, and teachers. One such source of support was Ida. She was the most gregarious, fiery, and opinionated seer I have ever known. I met Ida through one of my own clients, and she was a part of my family from that very first meeting. Ida was her own anomaly, unique and undefined. She was a seer through the ancient art of tasseography: she read coffee grinds, as did her mother before her. What stands out is that Ida would not allow anyone in her home to have their grinds read. You needed to have a car so your grinds could be read as you are parked in the vicinity with Ida at your side. She was forthright. As a client, you picked her up at the appointed time and drove a few blocks away to a location where you both felt comfortable. Then this elder seer would take out her blue rectangular tray, a large white plate to disseminate the coffee grinds on, and a little jar of water for washing the grinds away when she needed to see new formations on the plate. Ida was an experience for everyone to try. She loved spirits, particularly leprechauns, and the plant spirits loved her. I can tell because each time we walked past flowering plants, they seemed to bend her way.

During my current healing crisis, I knew I needed someone physical—in the earth plane—to help me. The work I had done in the cemetery had helped bring clarity to the souls involved, but also, since it cleared an energetic pattern in my own healing process, it had caused physical upheaval in my body. I needed Ida.

I made my way over to Queens on a bright autumn day to seek her assistance. We walked to my car; I carried her cornucopia of grounds-reading tools. She settled herself into my "talking car," as she always liked to call it. (She nicknamed it this because every time she said something the spirits approved of the car alarm would beep.)

Our favorite parking space was in a lot behind a local drugstore and our favorite pizzeria; we would pull in there and find a spot away from the other cars. Ida poured the Turkish coffee into the espresso coffee cup and I drank a little, since Ida wanted some of the coffee along with the grinds for the reading. If you have ever tried Turkish coffee, you know that it has a very dark and bitter taste—it's an acquired taste, at that.

Ida looked at the cup. She said there was a man standing there, a medicine man, a healer. She described him as having brown skin and a magic staff. I knew immediately that it was my shaman. She said that he was helping me and not to worry, for he was a good soul. She also saw that I was not feeling too well. She said that it was from a poison in my body, a poison that was trying to make its way out, slowly but surely.

She also saw negative spirits that were pestering me during the night. She told me not to worry, that they bother me because I'm a good soul and they would rather not see me get better. Whenever Ida saw souls like this, she would take her jar of water and just wash them away. But before she did that, a big cross appeared in one of the plates, visible even to my untrained eye. Ida looked at me and said that God was with me, so I should try and worry less.

We talked about a lot of other things that were helpful that day. Once in while a remedy would appear on the plate, or something about eating the right food or about some emotional upset I was focused on. Whatever it was, Ida brought healing to it. And just as it was with my shaman, I felt so much better when I left her presence.

As winter drew near and the cold humid weather seemed to project its tendrils into the city, I focused on the work I had learned with my shaman. My body was getting a little stronger each day, and I anxiously waited for the next piece of the puzzle to work with and integrate. The lost children continued to come. Even though some had crossed over, there were still what felt like hundreds stuck somewhere in the spirit world. I prayed for them daily, recounting the healings that the shaman and his helpers facilitated for me. Prayers and novenas to various Catholic saints would echo from my lips, and the children would continue to scatter about me and play with me from beyond the veil. Some of them really did not want to leave my company—and for that matter, I didn't want to lose theirs. Even so, I intuitively knew that one by one, they would someday go home, fully home.

The daylight grew shorter, and the holidays came upon us. I decided to enjoy some of the festivities and took a trip to the local zoo to see the Christmas lights. It was cold that night, and the sight of the illumined faces of children grasping their parents' hands was exhilarating. I felt like a child again. Whether we were forty years old or seven, we all looked with wonder at the lighted displays of Christmas magic. The petting zoo was open as well, and I enjoyed myself along with the kids, petting the farm animals. The night wouldn't have been complete without a hot pretzel, of course. It is rare for me to eat one, but I did so that night with joyous gluttony.

As I took my last bite of that salted, floury treat, I thought I saw my shaman out of the corner of my eye. I did a double take, and when he was nowhere to be found I thought it was my imagination. Over the past few weeks, I'd talked to him occasionally, but he seemed busy, and I knew that when the time was right he would reappear.

I walked toward the petting zoo again and watched the children climb up on the fences to touch whichever animal came closest to them. Their anticipation was overwhelming. I could feel how special it felt to be chosen by one of the animals, as the one whom the animal chose to commune with. After an animal made its choice, the other children would run over to the child who was "picked" to see if they could pet the animal too. This went on all night long. I even think the lost children followed me, because I could hear them laughing and giggling from the other side. They wanted to enjoy a bit of Christmas magic, too.

> Many of the talents and abilities we have been reserving for "higher" animals may in fact be part of the experience of all living things.
> In our attempts to understand the origin and nature of awareness, we ought to be looking far more closely, and more literally to our roots.
> — Lyall Watson

I finally left the petting zoo area and began walking down a narrow path that led to the camel exhibit. As I stopped by some flora that draped the pathway, I heard footsteps behind me, coming from the spirit world. They were gentle footsteps, watching me and protecting me. I knew the shaman was there. I'd had a few weeks to rest after our work with John and his relatives at the cemetery; my physical body needed that time to integrate, cleanse, and heal. My shaman was ready to continue the work, and I trusted that he knew I was ready, too.

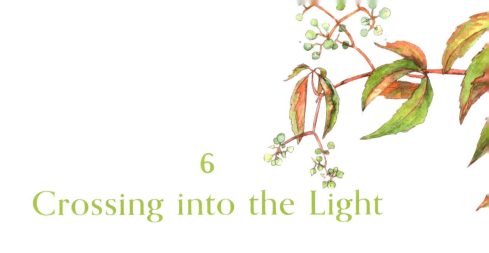

6
Crossing into the Light

The next day, in the midst of seeing clients, I knew with certainty that the shaman would soon come to show me the next piece of the puzzle. When he arrived later, he told me to go to the home of an acquaintance and do some spiritual cleansing there. Since I wasn't used to going into homes and cleansing them, I was a little hesitant about what my goal would be there.

The shaman explained that when I went into the home, I would see where some of the lost children came from. Years ago, the house had known abuse—spiritual, emotional, and mental. There had been four children living there, and all of them were very open to the spirit world. For some reason, the lost children who now surrounded me had attached themselves to them, as I'm sure they attached themselves to children all over the world who had similar spiritual patterns. I can't address the needs of the entire world, obviously, but it has always been my belief that when you help one, you help hundreds. When you help hundreds, you heal thousands. And when you heal thousands, a miracle happens. So numbers don't matter, because the efficacy of prayer moves mountains.

Before going to the house, I called my acquaintance (who knew a little about my work) and simply explained that I believed there were some stuck souls in his home; could I come in and pray? I told him that

I thought it would help his health as well. He was unbelievably fine with this proposal. I then went and bought some vanilla wafer cookies for the children, and some flowers. I also found a teddy bear I'd had since childhood.

The next day, when I walked into the house, I saw that it hadn't been cleaned in years. The walls were dilapidated and dirt hung from every corner—I almost walked out due to the scent of decay in there. It was sparsely furnished. I made my way through the house and into the smaller bedrooms. The girls used to sleep in one bedroom and their brother in another. Old posters and books were strewn across the floor and walls. I just looked around in disbelief for a while.

Finally, I took one of the chairs and lay the flowers on it. I got a bowl for the cookies and put some of the vanilla wafers in it. The teddy bear looked perfect sitting between the cookies and the flowers. As I walked through the house again, I called my shaman, and also kept talking to the lost children who had once lived there, letting them know that I was in a home they would probably recognize on some level. They wouldn't actually recognize the house as one they had occupied, but on a psychic level, they might perceive that it was a manifestation of an energy matrix they already knew, a physically manifested metaphor.

In the living room, I felt a portal between an old velvet-covered chair and a twenty-year-old TV set. What felt like a gust of wind went through me, opening my psychic vision wider. I could indeed see a wondrous portal awaiting the children. I was elated at the possibility of some continued healing for them. I went back into the bedroom and began to pray, knowing my shaman would be present when I needed him. I began with my rosary and then with the novenas that have always worked. I talked to the children in between the prayers. This was going to take more than one day—it would take a number of days and I would have to come back to this home often. I remember looking at the ceiling and saying to myself that the ceiling would collapse after the work was done.

I felt a presence behind me, which I assumed was my shaman. I turned around, and to my surprise it was John, the soul from the cemetery. He wanted to help in some way, and I began to truly understand how all things and souls connect. For some reason, it was his karma to help in the work. It didn't matter how; even just bringing me reassurance and extra protection was enough. I smiled and then continued praying. John was a humble and sweet presence, very different from the soul I'd originally encountered at the cemetery.

The energy and temperature in the room became frigid and I could vividly see the moisture in my breath. My body temperature also dropped, and my extremities became ice cold. The children became quiet for a while. I fervently repeated every word of every prayer, with the hopes that some of the children would see the portal and cross.

John stayed with me and when the time was right, my shaman appeared. The lost children still remained quiet—no laughing, no playing, no hide-and-seek. I comforted myself against the coldness of the air and felt some unusual presences. The orange-colored room was starting to feel more like a prison, and visions began coming to me of children from long ago. It seemed that many more lost children lived in this house than the four I'd been looking for. And these were visions I had not seen before—the energies startled me. These children were horrified; many of them had gone through some sort of ritualistic abuse. I also saw trains, many trains, and saw what looked like uniforms belonging to concentration camps. The energy of the abuse began to feel cultish in nature to me. I had a sense that some of the children in my visions were headed off to the concentration camps we read about in history books. Some of them had been kidnapped and suffered much. They all died in horror, some with chemical poisoning, others from starvation. I was petrified to be "seeing" all of this and really thought it couldn't be true. I felt a hand on my shoulder at one point—John, letting me know he was there with me.

I took a deep breath and wondered how it related to me, if at all. Then an idea dawned on me. The miasm—these souls must have been around my mom and presumably around my grandfather as well. Who knows how long they had been in my family's energy matrix. Both my mom and my grandfather had had those strange, near-death experiences. Since I don't know very much about my family history in the literal sense, I can only surmise that in some way, these children attached themselves to my family during those deathlike trances and were then passed on to me. The poisoning from the pesticides and what it did to my body had never made clinical sense. Why, for a year, did the skin on my body burn each night as I went to bed, making me writhe in pain between my blankets until it subsided? I could understand that an allergic reaction would cause that kind of sensation, but for so long a time was uncanny. Pieces of my puzzle were finally starting to fit; I was getting at least some understanding into the reasons behind the intensity of my health situation.

As I was integrating these pieces together, my body went into some sort of pain reaction. I continued to pray while figuring everything out. If I could make the connection between myself and these children, then it would be easier for them to cross over and for me to let go. Now that I realized how often they had been around my mother, I guessed that there had to have been a family ancestor who directly experienced some kind of trauma similar to what I was seeing. And in his or her quest to be free, the negativity surrounding that ancestor had taken hold of other family members, propelling them into that deathlike trance state.

The children were trying to free themselves, but they just didn't know how. My familial line was familiar to them, so they'd hung around for quite a while hoping someone would notice them. I still wasn't exactly sure why this house was chosen for this moment, or why some of those children's spirits were attached to the place, but I assume it had something to do with what went on with the children who'd lived there. Most likely, the children who lived there fragmented psychologically in some way due to the abuse they'd endured, and in their disconnect, they opened up to other planes of consciousness. I trust that the other young spirits attached to them to bring them some sort of comfort and relief.

> There is no death, only a change of worlds.
> Seattle, Suquamish Chief

There was no pragmatic answer here, but there were bits and pieces that could formulate a synopsis of what had transpired, energetically, over the last few generations in my family. After I left, I talked to the homeowner and got his okay for future visits—the days I'd planned to be there had just extended themselves.

My dreams became more lifelike over the next few days, as I could not escape the horrors that I'd seen and felt with those children's souls. I wasn't sleeping well. Part of that had to do with the fact that these new children were now around me more, and their pain had become mine until they could find solace. Emotionally, physically, and spiritually, we all seemed to be purifying at the same time.

My moods also began to change as I started working with this specific group of children. I isolated myself more and kept very few friends by my side. I talked with my mom often, but pretty much stayed disciplined in embracing the space that I needed to carry myself through this. Physically, my chemical sensitivities increased for a period of time. My sense of smell was so delicate and attuned, I was repelled by the scent of hair spray or perfume. My eyesight was out of focus—my vision would vacillate between nearsightedness and farsightedness. My energy field was so open that being near people became challenging. I was ornery. My appetite was unusual, as were my food cravings. My blood-sugar levels would rise and fall, and I was becoming increasingly food sensitive. And the body burning . . . every night, like clockwork, it would take its toll. I would clench my jaw so tightly that my mouth would hurt in the morning from grinding my teeth.

I saw my holistic practitioners as often as I could; they reflected on my need for extra protection and continued prayer. I also did a lot of work on my own. But I was getting tired—emotionally, physically, and spiritually. Even though the shaman had come into my life only a short time ago, I'd been working with the lost children for a while before that and fighting the pesticides in my body at the same time. I felt like I was lingering, suspended in some kind of spiritual animation. My priest had advised that whenever I took on a spiritual endeavor, I should always ask God if this is the work I should be doing. Go over and above the minds of the teachers in the spirit world, he said, and ask God. Well, I did ask God, over and over again. The answer was the same all the time.

One evening the body burning got really bad. The children were waiting for me to go back to the house a second time. A smell of fear and of dead animal carcasses permeated my house that evening. I kept looking at my herbs and my plants. I needed the shaman; I needed my plant god to distill his magic, because I was weak.

I drew a bath and asked the shaman what plants to put in it. I knew he would respond, and even though I couldn't see him this time, I could hear his answer clearly: "Rosemary and rue." I happened to have both of them on hand.

I took a handful of each and held them gingerly. Sometimes I just tossed plants into the bath; other times I steeped them and then poured the plant water in with the bathwater. I always prayed with my plants before bathing with them, however, and I wanted my shaman to pray with me, to energize and infuse the plants and the prayers with his magic, his gifts from the Creator.

I offered my prayers for both the rosemary and the rue—but not my usual prayers, because this time, I wanted to sing to the plants' souls, like my shaman did.

I pulled the rosemary toward my heart and began to sing its song:

O Divine Mother, all loving, all knowing, ever so present. Fill our hearts with the grace of your love. Hold us in your tender arms. Give to us divine mercy in our suffering. Be with us at the time of our loneliness. Show us how to be compassionate with ourselves and with humankind. Teach us the ways of God.

With that prayer, a little girl plant spirit came out of the ethers. She was transparent in nature, and very connected with the Divine Mother energy. She was filled with pure, unconditional love and had a special relationship with the plant world. She had her own garden in the ethers, and cared for all of her plants, especially rosemary. She was lovely as she whirled around me, psychically placing sprigs of rosemary in my hair. She told me not to worry, that I would be okay. She also said that the lost children would be okay too. She showed me that I would go back to their house soon, and that in the end, they would be fine. I placed the rosemary in my tub and knew that the energies imparted by both the little girl elemental and my shaman would make the bathwater strong.

The little girl danced her way back into the ethers, where I could only hear her gentle voice. My shaman's presence remained with me as I retrieved the rue, notably one of the most protective herbal plants there is. Just holding the rue made my body begin to feel better. I knew this bath was really going to help me. My extremities began to warm and my light-headedness started to dissipate. I had been so assiduous in taking care of my herbs that when I needed them, I trusted that they would be there for me. My muscles settled into a more relaxed position, and I placed the rue into the bathwater, laying some atop the floating rosemary. I looked into my heart for a prayer, and this is what fell from the sky onto my lips:

Almighty Spirit, bring us everlasting life as we embark on our journeys. Heal us from the ills of self and protect our souls from harm. We ask this in accordance with divine righteousness.

I echoed this prayer a few times. The vibration was so strong that I didn't know if I was going to be able to make a connection with the rue's elemental. I felt an intensity come through the ethers, but no elemental appeared. I thought I must have done something wrong and called out to the shaman to assist me. I waited patiently, and then, through the shaman's vision, I was able to see an energy. This energy was magnificent and had no form. It embellished the rue plant with its essence and stayed ensconced in the ethers so that its powers would remain strong.

There was a light glowing from the bathwater. I now could see my shaman, blessing it and also enhancing the powers of the elementals and the plants. That was his job. I stepped into the bath and allowed myself to partake in its healing energies for almost an hour. Over the following few days, I recuperated and my symptoms subsided gracefully. I knew I could soon head back to the house.

I started to frequent the home a few times each week, continuing to pray for the lost children. John showed up sometimes to support me. I eventually became stronger when I was there, and my body and spirit would be less affected each time I went. I would bring new cookies and new flowers on occasion, waiting until I knew the energy of the old cookies was eaten and the flowers withered. The energy of the home seemed to brighten with each visit, and my shaman watched over me whenever I went there. As time progressed, I was greeted by laughing children when I walked through the front door. The dead silence and heaviness began to change at the sound of this laughter. I was able to breathe better when I was there, and many of the child spirits were trusting me more. The portal in the living room seemed brighter each time, and souls would walk through it like it was any other opening. As the children healed, I knew that my time there was coming to an end. But it was not yet complete. I prayed, asking the shaman to help bring closure. This would be closure for these children, as well as mark a significant physical healing for myself. The miasm was continually being released and raised to the light, and my ancestors were also being freed.

The energies that had not allowed me to heal in entirety before were now weakened, and the spirits that we (my spirit guides and I) had been helping thus far were playing an integral part in that.

I prepared myself to go into the house one last time. I sat on my living room floor with my rosebud beaded rosary and meditated. I asked the shaman and the plant world, along with all the saints I pray to, to give me guidance.

As I was praying, I felt a tapping on my shoulder. I turned to see the spirit of an elderly lady. She told me she was a storyteller, a wise woman, who loved to create pottery. She surrounded herself with children, or rather, they followed her wherever she went. She told them stories, and they listened with fervor and never left her side. She showed me that she was the guardian (plant spirit) of the sage plant, and that she would come with me to the house and walk the remainder of the children into the light—those who wanted to go and were ready to go. She asked me to prepare some sage for our journey. I did so immediately.

I drove over to the house with my tools and what felt like a carload of spiritual helpers. The children always knew when I was coming. I loved coming to that house now. It was joyful.

My shaman was already there, and I could see John out of the corner of my eye, a smile on his face. I'd brought some more cookies and set them down on the floor. This felt like a celebration. The elderly woman, the storyteller, was at my side. I sat and went into a meditative space as the woman began to tell stories. The children gathered near her one by one, curious, to listen. They held on to her gray woolen skirt, whose train seemed to travel miles on the etheric floor.

In the background was my shaman. He silently lowered his head and breathed his prayer. He indicated that I should gather my sage and bring it forward to the middle of the room. With one breath, he breathed a prayer to imbue the sage and the elderly woman with the intensity of powers they had never known before. He was benevolent, merciful toward the child spirits.

Grandmother, we open our arms to take in your wisdom. Let us not be foolish in our ways. Heal us from impatience and ignorance. Help us to walk the path of righteousness with Spirit. Guide us and help us to guide those who come after us. We pray to you, O Grandmother, that we may be made humble and pass on your wisdom.

I watched. The shaman sang those words with ardor. And the elderly woman distilled her storytelling magic. The auras around the children became lighter, and my body was starting to beam. The energetic cords that had been attaching the children and myself were falling apart, and my physical and energetic bodies were lighter. We were in the midst of splendor, and the home had never felt so enchanting.

Having received her blessings from the shaman and the Creator, the elderly woman gently picked up the train of her woolen skirt from the floor. The children held on with all their being. She walked through the living room, glancing at the children with a smile. Never once halting the magical words of her story, she took them gracefully through the portal. The aroma of the sage plant filled the air, and even the cookies seemed to be acknowledged as their life-force was taken. The house began to quiet as the last of the child spirits walked through that portal. I turned to see where my shaman was. He had already departed.

I sat in the room for a moment, by myself, still on the floor. I just looked around. The room was neither empty nor full—it just was there. I didn't hear any laughter or crying. I actually didn't hear anyone talking to me or connecting with me from the other side. It was as though what had just transpired had never taken place.

I picked up my belongings and went home.

I slept well over the next few days. My body was healing, and my spirit was elated. I called the owner of the home to let him know that I no longer needed to come to his house anymore. He told me that a few days after I was last there, part of the bedroom ceiling had collapsed. I had predicted as much. The energy matrix for the lost children was broken, and I trusted that it was also broken for myself. Now it was time for me to heal those broken cords and undo some of the chaos that had been done. I had not been able to break the pattern before I met the shaman, but for some reason, this was all meant to happen the way in which it did.

During my morning meditations, some of the children would continue to pass by to say hello. But they were no longer stuck. They came by just to let me know they missed me and that they were doing fine.

I felt freer inside and ready to learn more from my shaman about his work with plant spirit healing. He let me know that sometime soon we would visit the countryside and do more work with souls and plants. That is where I would learn most of what I needed to know about his plant spirit magic. Until that time, however, he wanted me to focus on practicing with my clients what I had learned so far and also on repairing my health at a cellular level—the pesticides were ready to exit my nervous and immune systems. I knew that he was right; through seeing clients, my own healing process would continue.

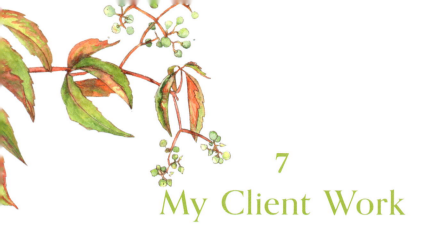

7
My Client Work

Becky

Becky called me one day to schedule a session. I had never met her before. When she arrived for her appointment, I saw that she was a beautiful, middle-aged European woman who was struggling with asthma and bronchitis. She worked as a nurse and was happily married with a few children. She was very devout and prayed often, but the nagging cough and wheezing persisted. I did an intake and learned that she used an inhaler when necessary but wasn't fond of allopathic medicine and its focus on drugs and surgery. I asked about her family history; she said that her mother was also a pious woman who prayed reverently, and that for some reason she suspected that it was her relationship with her mother that was tying her into her health condition. I communicated with the other side and passed along the information I'd received during the intake, for confirmation.

Becky was relieved by our conversation—someone finally understood her. As we talked, I found that I kept shaking my head and dropping it toward one side, so I asked her who'd had the stroke in her family. Her father had, and he'd survived. Then my lungs became suffused with smoke and I couldn't breathe, so I was curious about which relative was the smoker. Her mother was. As I opened the door to her relatives in the spirit world, it seemed like I was in the middle of a family gathering. I was emphatically picking up various symptoms that my client shared with relatives on the other side. For some reason, her ancestors had decided to make their way into her energy field and finish their earthly work through Becky without her permission. No wonder she was having so many headaches!

I needed to figure out Becky's relationship with these ancestors to discover where this pattern had started. After talking some more, I found out that her mother, Maria, who was very involved in family matters, had allowed the family to really bulldoze their way into her life and the lives of those immediately around her. This had made her mother sickly and emotionally weak; she felt powerless against the busybodies in the family and didn't have a voice. No one seemed to pay attention to Maria—they just told her what to do all the time. Her addiction to cigarettes had helped her deal with some of her anxieties.

When Maria got married, she married into the same pattern. Her husband didn't respect her and yelled at her all the time. Maria was not a fighter. She would cry often and run to church and pray. When she had children, she kept them close. She protected them but needed their protection as well. Emotional boundaries were confusing for Maria and her children; she sought out her children as confidants at times. Becky, who was the oldest girl, was the most confused of all the children. Because of Maria's insecurities, she'd inadvertently used Becky as an emotional and energetic shield. Even at age four, Becky would argue and defend her mother if anyone in the family treated her badly. She could feel, even so young, the energy of someone hurting her mother. More importantly, she was able to experience her mother's pain. Becky grew up like this until, in her early twenties, she left home and likewise married young. Luckily she married an emotionally healthy man, but she took on the health and spiritual issues that her family had placed upon her. One of her children even energetically inherited the lung weakness, which developed into repetitive bronchitis.

I needed to work with Becky on developing the proper boundaries. I also needed to work with her ancestors on the same thing. It was also important that Becky express some unresolved grief and anger from her childhood, and that would take some time.

The first thing I wanted to do was give Becky an ally—a plant ally—that she could call upon. Through prayer, she could activate the cellular memory of the plant's healing energies. I felt the energy of my shaman in the ethers; he was present just for support if I needed it. I told Becky that I would ask my guides for an ally for her, and then she could learn how to be in relationship with it.

I held her hand and prayed, and gold energy filled my psychic vision. Off in the distance, I saw what appeared to be a Catholic saint. How perfect, since Becky and her family were devout Catholics. I looked closer and saw that it was St. John the Baptist—and then I knew that the plant he was holding for Becky was St. John's wort.

I heard my prayer in my heart and began to speak its words:

Divine Truth, shed for us healing waters through your many tears. Shed for us the breath of life through your blood. Deliver us into the grace of eternal life. Grant us peace within.

The energy of those words surrounded Becky until she felt a calm come over her. She sensed a lightness around her, and I told her it was the energy bestowed by St. John's wort.

I prayed to the shaman, too, and asked him to bless the healing session. What happened next was similar to what I'd experienced when my shaman first conducted a healing on me: not only did elementals from the plant world appear, but anointed ones in the spirit world who had the capacity to intensify the healing effect of plant spirit medicine also made their presence known. They seemed to like Becky very much and wanted to help her feel better. The elementals seemed to be whirling around her, while the shaman, along with another medicine man trained in Eastern healing arts and a Native American healer, graced the room we were sitting in. All I had done was open up the space for these beings to come and assist. I watched as all who were present worked on the issues Becky was struggling with.

Becky coughed a little, and as the work was being done, she began to talk about her childhood and her mother. She loved her mother immensely. She remembered her mom and dad yelling all the time and how, after a while, her mother just gave up fighting. It wasn't worth it to her, and she began to withdraw from conflict and internalize her anger. Becky had watched as her mother was criticized and cast away by various family members. When Becky asked her mom why the family was so mean to her, Maria couldn't give her an answer. From the time Becky was young and her mom seemed to give up, she became Maria's voice and protected her. As Becky got older, her father was hard on her as well, but her mom failed to defend her when Becky felt she needed it. But Becky had a voice and was a fighter.

Tears were rolling down Becky's face as she relayed these memories to me, and her breathing became a little hampered. She started to have a panic attack, so I told her to recall the energy of the beginning of the session when I'd prayed and she'd felt calm. She did so, and with that, the gold light and some of the beings appeared to reinforce what she needed. Becky could feel this, even though she wasn't able to see what was going on.

She waited a few minutes until her panic subsided and then continued to recall her painful past. She remembered one experience in particular: once, when she was a teenager, she came home past her curfew and her father went into a rage. Her mother actually tried to defend her, but to no avail—her father was stronger. Becky was angry with her mother for not being as powerful as her father and said that it was that way for her most of her life. She wept, not just for herself, but for her mom.

After all these years, she was still carrying her mother. This was evident when Maria's spirit appeared behind her. Although Maria was still alive at the time, her spirit was able to join us in that moment. It came through as both her higher self and her lower self. When Becky was recalling the trauma of her childhood, I could see Maria in the background, crying and hiding in the corner of my vision. In spirit, she appeared to be a pale and unnerved woman. Her life-force was diminished. That was her lower self—the part of her that was still stuck in the past somehow and could not let its trauma be healed.

When Becky could finally release and have a good cry and affirm her love for her mother, Maria's higher self appeared. She came in much lighter and brighter at that point. Her face was soft and filled with compassion and concern for her daughter. She energetically filled the room with hugs for Becky in the hopes that Becky could feel them. I was working with Becky's spirit in the hope that she could reconcile with that part of herself that felt loved, safe, and powerful, all the while invoking the St. John's wort healing magic.

It was important for me to work with Maria, too, so that the negativity that caused her soul to be stuck could be undone—and so that eventually she could let go of Becky. Becky also needed to let go of her mom when the time was right. We talked about that at length, and Becky had much homework to do. Her grief and rage were at times immeasurable, so I suggested that she start a journal while remembering to call upon the healing energies of St. John's wort, which we'd invoked at the start of the session. Writing would help her express what she could not express verbally. Becky left with an abundance of things to do before we met again. I knew that the energy of St. John's wort would stay with her until she no longer needed it.

When Becky came back a few weeks later, she was lighter. She mentioned that she and her mom went out to dinner one evening and enjoyed themselves; Becky remarked that her mom was a bit different, as if a small amount of weight had been taken off her shoulders. She was keeping a journal, and we looked it over. Becky read me passages that embraced the past, the present, and her hopes for the future. She'd talked mostly about her mom in the early entries and then started to focus on herself. She told me she would meditate and remember to ask the St. John's wort to be present and try to allow herself to receive the same energies that she had experienced during our first time together. Becky was on her way to healing.

We met a number of times over the next year. Becky was growing stronger in herself, developing better boundaries with her mother and taking better care of herself. She enrolled in some art classes and focused on simply eating better and exercising. Little by little, she was letting go of her mom, and little by little, her health was improving. She began to become aware of the times when her asthma and bronchitis were triggered and did her best to try to heal it. She was able to bring herself into a meditative space more easily as the time passed and grew accustomed to always being surrounded by healing energies. To her surprise, she found herself enjoying the time she spent with her mother, not feeling burdened anymore by her mother's emotions.

Becky was now able to see her mom as separate from herself and worked effortlessly to have compassion for her from a different place within. After we stopped meeting, I heard that Becky was enjoying her life to the fullest and continuing to take very good care of herself. I also heard that her mother passed, and I knew that both Becky and Maria were now free.

Robert

Robert walked into my Connecticut office in the wintertime. The first time we met turned out to be a very interesting session. He supposedly came because his physicians had diagnosed him with early rectal cancer, but he wanted to talk about many other things. The cancer was the last thing on his mind that day.

Mainly, Robert wanted to know all there was to know about God and the angels. I was stupefied. He literally had a list of questions; the first was whether God loved him and how I knew that. He also wanted to know if God forgave him for all the mistakes he'd made in his life. I knew at that point that Robert was going to be a special client, and indeed he was. It turns out he had a wife and children and loved them dearly. He was also very passionate about his work and enjoyed his life very much. But despite all that, he was carrying around a deep-seated sense of self-rejection. He smoked marijuana often, in small hits, so that he could try to open up to those states of consciousness that he was now asking me about.

> If a man would pass through Paradise in a dream, and have a flower presented to him as a pledge that his soul had really been there, and if he found that flower in his hand when he awoke—Aye! and what then?
> *Samuel Taylor Coleridge*

Robert and I spent all of that first session talking about God. Messages came through from the other side regarding his life, his thoughts, his dreams. Robert needed a lot of convincing that God loved him. He asked me if I thought God was angry about his mistakes. I told him that God loved him and wasn't angry in the way that he perceived he was. It was like Robert was trying to prove, to himself and to me, that he was unworthy of any kind of unconditional love from a higher power. He believed that his family and friends loved him, but he could not believe in a God who loved him.

As our conversation progressed, I sensed that Robert had a lot of rage toward his father. He'd mentioned briefly that his dad was very controlling and wanted him to be perfect. Robert had pursued his father's affections and approval for most of his life, but never seemed to get it. He often felt judged, and this affected the way he lived in the world. I could tell that he feared masculine energy and ended up rebuking it within himself. He couldn't assimilate love of self and love from a higher power. Because he viewed God as a masculine energy (as opposed to a feminine one), he accepted the notion that he was unable to receive or be worthy of any kind of love from above. He felt like he existed without form at times.

Robert spent his life testing himself, testing God, and testing all the masculine relationships in his life. Feminine relationships were manageable for him—for the most part he enjoyed his female friendships and adored the women in his family. He was allowing feminine energy to dominate his masculine side, so there was an unhealthy balance.

Robert didn't want to explore his past in too much detail, since he felt there was no need to at the time. I was brief on the topic, just mentioning offhand how some of his relationship with his dad played a role in how he related to himself. Robert wasn't ready to hear that, nor did he have any interest in it. He just wanted to focus on his relationship with God.

I did the best I could during our hour. Robert had a quizzical look on his face whenever I spoke. When our time was done, he thanked me graciously and left the office. I wasn't sure what to make of our meeting, so I left it at that.

A year passed, and I didn't hear back from Robert until he called to schedule another appointment, asking if I remembered him. Of course I did; I said I would be happy to work with him again.

When he walked into my office, he seemed angry. He was angry with me, with everyone, with God. He asked why, at our previous meeting, I hadn't seen or told him that his cancer would progress rapidly and that his prognosis would be grim. After all, I was an intuitive medium and I should have known that. I responded by saying that I understood he was angry and that when he came to see me a year ago, he hadn't wanted to discuss the cancer during the session. Furthermore, even if he'd wanted to, I'm not God and cannot see everything when a person comes to me. No medium or psychic can.

At this point, Robert's cancer had spread farther into his intestinal tract and liver. He had undergone a few surgeries and was also going through chemotherapy. He looked desperate and destitute of spirit. When I looked into his eyes, I saw defiance—defiance toward God and toward his inner knowing—a power struggle. It was all part of the process he was working through. When I asked him why he had come back, he said he wanted to talk more about God. Once again, he wanted to feel God loving him, to know that God loved him. And significantly, he wanted to look at how his father had made him feel all of his life.

I thought we should begin by talking about his dad in a little more depth. I asked him to help me understand his father in his own words. Michael, Robert's dad, was a retired military man. He and his wife had only one child and settled in a suburb in western New York. Michael was not a hands-on dad, so to speak. It was Robert's mom who reared him for most of his life and gave him the emotional nourishment he needed. Michael was a very silent man for the most part, which was how he controlled Robert. Whenever he spoke with Robert, it was to criticize him for something that had just occurred; he would not say anything at all if Robert was looking for some feedback. Michael was an empty soul, and Robert did whatever he could to gain his approval, as opposed to silence or a few words of disdain.

Robert thought it was his fault that he was never acknowledged or received by his father. Although his mother saw what was going on and tried to distract him to make him feel better, this only served to increase and validate Robert's growing anger. He spent most of his young and early adult life living this pattern. His way of dealing with it was the marijuana that he'd started smoking at a pretty young age. He wanted to know if he'd caused his cancer. I told him no, and I was not going to let him use that as an excuse to further punish himself for not being "good enough."

I had my work cut out for me—Robert was convinced that he was unworthy of love and healing. It wasn't time to work with plant medicine yet, since I felt we needed to make him a little stronger first. I went over his diet with him, and suggested some nutrition, supplementation, and strengthening and detoxification techniques that he could do at home. Robert was already seeing a number of holistic practitioners as well as allopathic medical doctors. He wanted to get as much support and information as he could to help him on his journey. He had a therapist, acupuncturist, holistic medical doctor, and various other healing artists. He would even talk about them in session and ask me if I thought they were helping him. I would reply by asking him if *he* thought they were.

Robert scheduled sessions with me every two weeks. We kept to that schedule until the day he died, three years later. We worked slowly, and through our sessions, continued to explore his family dynamics and relate them to how he saw himself in this world. For the first few months, although he left every session thanking me, he wasn't sure if the sessions were helping at all. Although he didn't know if he believed in anything I said, he returned time after time. Each time, he told me that he'd done what I'd suggested, as well as followed the advice of his numerous other practitioners. But he couldn't tell if any of it was making a difference.

Then there was a session, a few months after we'd started, when Robert walked in with a gleam in his eye. I asked him what was different. He said something had begun to shift within him, and he thought he was beginning to feel the presence of God around him. I asked how he knew. He said he'd started to feel a calm in his heart and wanted more. He felt a serenity about him at times when things were chaotic, and he didn't know where it was coming from. He wanted to feel and know this energy in every aspect of his life and wanted to try to garner more of this higher power. What he didn't realize was that this power had been within him all along. But Robert still wasn't ready for a plant spirit—I wanted to do some work with his father first.

During one session, I had Robert on the table for some hands-on energy and cranial work. I asked him to think about his father and tell me about events from his childhood that he still held resentment about. He didn't need to tell me aloud; I just wanted to observe his energy body and see what reaction his father's spirit would have. As Robert started to visualize these childhood stories in his head, his energy field shifted and his organs pulsed rapidly. His eyelids were flickering back and forth, and he twitched on the massage table. I looked over my shoulder as I felt his father's spirit draw near. I asked, telepathically, what his father wanted from him and why he wouldn't let Robert go.

Michael proceeded to tell me that he loved his son but had been very disappointed in him ever since he could remember; that it felt like no matter what Robert did, Michael was aware that he could not connect with his son on the level he wanted to. I asked Michael about his relationship with his own father, and he showed me pictures of a similar relationship, one in which his own father disowned him. This was something that Michael had never gotten over, and since he never rooted himself in a healthy paternal relationship with his own dad, he did not have the tools or the desire to do so with his own son. He grieved because he realized he had nothing to offer Robert. When I asked him again why he was holding on to his son, he said it was the only way he was able to deal with his feelings about his own father. Michael knew that Robert carried a lot of anger toward him—Robert had vented it from time to time. And while Robert had at least had some opportunity to express his anger at his father, Michael, having been disowned, had not. Through Robert, Michael was able to have some sort of connection with his own dad, a sort of emotional incest if you will. I talked with Michael while my hands were still working on the back of Robert's head; Robert fell into a gentle sleep.

I asked Michael if he wanted to learn how to relate to his own feelings, and if he wanted his son to be free of some pain. He said yes. I told him that while my focus was on his son, I would give him some tools to help him on his journey.

I called in my shaman and asked him to help. I asked him to guide me to the best plant medicine to help with this family dynamic. The room became still, with Robert still in a sleep/dreamtime space. My breathing became labored for a few moments, then cleared, and an energy seemed to whirl up the front of my body and into my head, making me dizzy. I heard myself mumbling some syllables—magical syllables. I knew a plant prayer and invocation were coming.

Rod of light, cast down upon us your invincible power of God. Through the Holy Spirit, manifest the truth of all things hidden and unseen.

My voice grew deeper and louder, and I repeated the prayer.

Rod of light, cast down upon us your invincible power of God. Through the Holy Spirit, manifest the truth of all things hidden and unseen.

I've never inhaled and exhaled so deeply in my life. With my shaman present, Robert still in twilight, and Michael's spirit hovering, another spirit approached our space.

It was a male soul who had lived on earth hundreds of years ago and was somehow connected to the plant kingdom. When he died, he apparently left a number of issues in his life uncompleted. He'd walked the earth's gardens in spirit for centuries, and one of the plants he'd befriended, along with its elementals, was the skullcap. The elementals loved this soul and literally took him under their wings. He'd received much comfort from them and seemed to make nature, especially the skullcap plant, his new home. It was his own heaven. He took care of the gardens he came across and made a vow to assist others in bringing completion to their life stories. Between the earth's spiritual gardens and the clouds, he kept himself pretty busy—heaven's gardener, of sorts.

This spiritual gardener appeared to be very joyful and light of soul, and he took Michael by his energy field and danced around. He showed

Michael his gardens, and then led him down memory lane, showing him scenes of the arguments Michael had had with Robert, and how they'd both felt afterward. Michael was saddened by the memories, but the gardener pressed on. He wanted Michael to begin to acknowledge some of his own pain. As always, what felt like hours took only minutes in real time. Then he led Michael back to his garden and brought him near the skullcap. He transmitted the energy of the skullcap onto Michael's spirit, which began to cry. The skullcap was able to penetrate some of the emotional wall that had built up.

Michael looked at his son Robert, still sleeping on my table, and compassion filled his eyes. The gardener and Michael then exchanged some words that I couldn't hear, and the gardener left. I saw the gleam still in Michael's eye and asked him if he was ready to let his son go. He said yes. I wished him well as he disappeared into the ethers.

Robert seemed to be waking. He didn't realize that he'd fallen asleep. He said he'd dreamt something about his father but couldn't remember what. He got up from the table and said he felt that presence again, that calm in his heart. When he thought about his father, he didn't feel as enraged as before.

Weeks turned into months and months turned into years. Robert and I continued to do work about his father, and I would psychically call in the skullcap plant to assist Robert when he was stuck. I didn't tell him about the healing energies of this plant but used it whenever he took a step back. If it was good for his father, and the relationship with his dad was the source of the original wounding, then I knew the skullcap would also benefit Robert and protect him when his father's lower self would come in—if it did at all.

Robert was healing, and I was elated. He seemed freer than he ever had in his life and was learning to detach himself in a healthy way from the traumatic memories of his past. He also learned, over the years we worked together, to have compassion for himself and forgive himself for what he thought he'd contributed to the abusive relationship. His stride came back, and he felt confident that his cancer would be healed. I knew only that his spirit was healing, as was the pattern that had helped create his malady—but I reserved judgment on the progression of his cancer, as I always felt that it was between him and God.

Our sessions were varied, and we began to focus more on Robert's life as a whole, not just his childhood. One day, Robert came to me and said he wanted to stop the chemotherapy and the cancer-fighting drugs he was on. He had been through so many treatments and had had chemotherapy on and off for years. Now that he felt emotionally so much freer, he wanted to be free of the disciplined regime of cancer fighting as well. He asked me what I thought, and I told him that I couldn't make that decision for him. He understood and said that he needed to go with his gut. So he stopped all forms of allopathic treatment and decided to continue with only a handful of holistic practitioners, me being one of them. He even took a break from our sessions for a month or so, and then came back. He just needed some time to have fun, as much as his body would let him. Robert deteriorated quickly after stopping his previous regime. I had a feeling he knew that he would. I got a call from him saying that he didn't think he had long now. He was immobilized in a hospital bed in a hospice, with the tender care of nurses and his family by his side. I went to see him. His skin seemed shrunk down to his bare bones, and flesh hung from every wasting muscle. But I didn't focus on that—I only focused on the bright light around him. I asked how he was doing, and he said he was okay. To my surprise, he asked again if God loved him. I told him, unequivocally, yes. I saw the spirits of his ancestors in the room and let him know that they would be there when he was ready to cross, and that even though he was afraid, he would not be alone. I promised him that it would not be as frightening as he expected, and that as he got closer, he would begin to see all the spirits I saw and simply leave his body and walk with them. I asked him if there was anything else he needed from me, and he said he wanted me to make sure his family was okay afterward. I told him I would do that.

I knew that now, at last, was the time to offer Robert plant magic to help his transition. We had worked together for so long that he'd gotten used to my quirkiness. I meditated for a moment, and gently said the prayer that came to me.

We call on you, ancestors of the earth and sky. Hear our prayers. We thirst for wholeness. We hunger for nourishment. And when we are ready to come home to the Great Spirit in the sky, carry us on your wings and fly.

Robert laughed, as he always did if he thought my work was too esoteric. But being the amazing sport that he always was, he went with it. His curiosity still intact, he inquired as to which spirit I was calling in now. He knew I worked with plant medicine, so he was not totally in shock when I said that I was calling on a plant for him and wanted him to call upon it himself during his transition, whenever he felt afraid. He was okay with the proposition. I laughed with him and echoed my prayer again. Then I saw, upon the bare white walls of his hospice room, a medicine man. He was chanting and holding a piece of mugwort in his hand. He was perched on a rock over a blazing fire. I stared at the fire for a bit and, interestingly enough, Robert said he started to feel some warmth come over his body—he thought it had something to do with what I was working with. I hadn't told him of the vision yet. I watched as the medicine man drew the plant to his mouth and forehead, each time reiterating prayers for the earth and for those who were dying. His special gift involved assisting souls in crossing over. I wanted to respect his space and was not intrusive. I pulled my energy back from the vision and humbly asked that this spirit be there for Robert when he needed him. I did not get an answer, but I knew that I was heard, and I had faith that my request would be honored.

I turned to Robert and told him what I'd experienced. He laughed again. I knew I would be hearing that laugh for the last time. I instructed him to call upon the mugwort plant and also the vision as he remembered it through my experience. I said that every time he did, he would feel as peaceful as he did now. We actually laughed some more. I gave him a hug goodbye and told him I would check in with him to see how he was doing when he got to the other side.

As I walked out of the room, I wanted to burst into tears. But I remained composed, since I needed to spend a few minutes with his family.

Robert crossed over a few days later. He was still laughing. I could hear it echoing through the heavens.

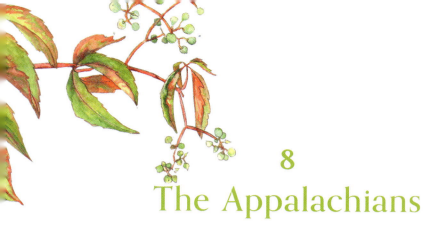

8
The Appalachians

In addition to utilizing my new plant healing knowledge to help clients, I continued to practice my work in other ways as well. It proved to be an invigorating privilege bestowed upon me by the spirit world. My body had gained much of its strength back and the miasm was almost completely healed.

Summertime was upon us, and I wanted to plant some of the plants that kept popping into my mind. I had a very small plot of land behind my home, not enough for a big garden, but enough for me to plant the thirty or so plants I kept thinking about.

I took a trip to an herbal gardening store in Connecticut and picked up some of what I needed. I ordered some of the more exotic annuals online. I cleared my soil and nourished it. I didn't leave much room in between my plantings; in my excitement, I had overestimated how much space I really had. After planting the seedlings, I smudged my garden. I sat there every day for two weeks and smudged, prayed, and even sang songs, using my rattle for accompaniment (living as I did in a tight-knit suburb of New York City, I knew my neighbors would think I was nuts, but I didn't care). My sister came to visit when I was putting the seedlings in the ground, and when she visited again two weeks later, the seedlings had literally grown over a foot. She was astonished and asked them what kind of miracle plant food I had given them. I told her that I'd smudged with sage, prayed, and rattled. She just laughed and said no more.

I knew that these plants were going to be the basis for a book I would write, and that later on, I would be spiritually journeying with the plants I had grown, asking for the healing remedies they could offer. It was one thing to always have been given remedies by the spirit world; it was another to be invited in—by the plant kingdom and the plant gods—as a conduit for another type of healing work. I was excited, even more so than before. I would be able to put their healing magic into words and share them with others.

I continued to nourish my plants until it was time for the next piece of my work to begin. The first leg of this spiritual journey took me to the foothills of the Appalachian Mountains. My shaman had told me that some of the work we would be doing would involve actual traveling, and that some of the remedies would be dispensed in mountainous countryside. And thus it came to be.

That summer, circumstances led me to over two hundred acres of unspoiled land. I was to spend a week there immersed in nature. The pine trees endlessly traversed the hills, and the presence of ancient spirits was obvious. Many could still hear their footsteps, and their imprints were the breath of the land. The oaks stood tall and majestic, unwavering at my delight upon arrival. I could actually feel their excitement as golden rays of sunlight poured down onto their branches. Out of the corner of my eye, I spotted a great horned owl hovering above, as though it knew I was coming and was watching my every move.

During the day, the air was warm and sultry. The nights were cool and awe-inspiring. I slept well the first night I arrived, awaking at the crack of dawn to begin my work. I took a journal with me, my rattle, some sage and other protective herbs, and gifts for the spirit world. I hadn't a clue where to begin, so I kept vigil as those in the spirit world guided me to the ground that I would pray upon.

I sat in the middle of a lustrous, overgrown hillside, the grass almost as tall as I was. There was no other human being around. But every living creature knew I was there, and every spirit knew as well. I took my tools from my satchel and began to pray. I went into a deep meditative space and my psychic vision became very refined. I told the spirits of the land why I was there—that I was meant to learn more about plant medicine and be of service if they needed me. I had to gain their trust and realized it wasn't going to be easy.

I looked around as I prayed and began to get glimpses of times past. I saw animals, mostly deer, that had starved to death on that land. They were running around in spirit, their bodies emaciated and malnourished, searching desperately for food. This took me aback a little, as I was not used to seeing animal spirits this way. Then the visions started to become clearer. Bloodshed—war between the Native Americans and the white men—and women and children lost and frightened. I could not forget the sight of the women and children (throughout my time in the mountains, they were perhaps the friendliest). I didn't see the medicine men or warriors at first; the male spirits of the land seemed to stay clear of me at the beginning, until I could prove my worthiness.

> We don't see things as they are.
> We see things as we are.
>
> *Anaïs Nin*

I stayed on the hillside throughout the afternoon, taking notes on what I was observing. Some of the Native children had been left motherless, and some of the mothers were left without their children. This reminded me of some of the lost children I had worked with. My shaman was somewhere in the ethers, but this was not his territory. He respected the domain of other souls and had pulled his energy back from me.

The friends I was staying with told me of a plot of land where they had tried in earnest to cultivate vegetation, but to no avail. That first afternoon, I walked over to that ground and saw that it was sacred. There had been mass killings of women and children on that parcel, and their souls continued to wander.

I wasn't too happy about what I had seen that first day and could only wonder what the rest of my trip would bring. I decided one of the first things to do was to ask my friends if they had any extra food for the deer spirits that had starved on that land. They did, and the next afternoon we took a walk, throwing the food down and letting the deer spirits know it was solely for them. I let my friends continue to do that while I tried to make contact with some of the women and children I'd seen. I sat and thought about the best way to approach this, remembering my lost children who had crossed over. I called upon them, any of them, to come and assist me. In just moments, pieces of my hair were being pulled and, oh, their laughter was so contagious and memorable. I asked them to befriend the children that I was seeing here, to play with them. While they did that, I focused on befriending the women.

Surrounded by all the native flora, I put on my gloves and carefully harvested a handful of nettles growing near me. I held it up to my heart and started to hum. The humming came so easily, as sparrows circled above and butterflies fluttered about with their dew-drenched wings.

O loving kindness, drench the fires of our bitterness and scorn. Weep not, for the ills of the human heart can only be appeased by your unbounded gracious love.

My heart expanded with love for the nettles and, obviously, for the women and children I was seeing. I waited with anticipation for the plant elemental or deva to appear, and lo and behold, tickling my ear were two delightful fairies. I wasn't expecting fairies in the midst of all this wounding, but there they were, bright and bold. They were radiating love, gentleness, tenderness, all of the feelings that were channeling through me. These fairies were supporting one another, exchanging healing energies one at a time and glowing in response to the gifts being offered. I just went with it, in the hopes that the souls of these women and children would see the fairies and come closer to me. I truly needed to leave this in God's hands.

I played with the fairies. They frolicked around me, and my lost children knew to come near. They had already befriended some of the Native children and motioned them to come over to where the fairies were playing. As in earth reality, if a child wanders, a mother will follow. Even though some of the Native children in the spirit world were motherless, the other mothers took care of them. When the mothers and children had died, trauma had caused some of their souls to become stuck in some unidentifiable dimension of the spirit world, while the others had indeed managed to cross into the light and, with tireless effort, were trying to reunite with their loved ones.

The lost children dallied a bit, until they knew that the Native children's souls were behind them, and then one and all danced around the pine tree. I said hello to the Native children and then just sat where I was, so as not to frighten them. The mothers came over and looked at me from a few yards away. I smiled gently and wanted them to know I was no threat to them. Spirits are always curious when someone on this side of the veil can see them.

I kept the tone of my voice gentle while I told them that I would do what I could to help them. I said I didn't know how yet, but I had been led there to do some work and, prayerfully, the guides who helped me thus far would support my endeavors on behalf of the souls wandering that land. I wondered, though, if I had overstepped my bounds, because I knew there were literally thousands of souls on that land. I only saw hundreds by the time I left, but I felt certain that thousands were lost. I was befuddled. I had been in that place before, not knowing why I was where I was or what I was supposed to do about it. But I watched as the women and children took care of one another, and they watched me. I left them in peace, telling them I would be back the next day to talk with them.

I felt a little relieved that evening before going to bed. I'm not sure why, exactly. I guess I felt I was making some headway, even though I still had no precise direction.

I was ravenous the next morning and cooked a hearty breakfast. I went out into the fields early to find my new acquaintances. The women and children were out, and they were playing. My lost children were still there as well, and even more fairies were fluttering around. I looked at the deer spirits. They didn't look as emaciated as they did when I'd first arrived, and their coloring was a little better (as best as one can perceive coloring on the other side of the veil). That made my heart warm. I sat with my journal and my rattle and thought I would start out by working with some of the plants growing around me. I'd assumed that the main reason I was there was to gather medicinal and spiritual information about some of the plants I would use for my book, while also knowing that if I was going to help any spirits, this would be the way to do it.

I wanted to embrace every living thing and every soul near me. I wanted to feel the strength of the pine tree roots reaching far into the unadulterated earth. I wanted to soar like the red-tailed hawks that encircled the sky above me. I wanted to shine in the brilliant sun like the dainty flowers of the chamomile plant. I wanted to be a part of everything around me. In seeing how hungry the deer were, how frightened the Native children seemed, the desperation those mothers of long ago still carried in their souls, I needed to somehow reconcile the beauty I was beholding before me with the wounds of the past I was also seeing. I begged the medicine spirits of the land to help me, to show me a way to embrace the world that they had known, and to let me offer, through my prayers, any solace that might be obtained.

I always knew that the only power there is comes from God. The privilege that we all receive is the privilege to pray, and to do so abundantly. The gift I was given before birth was to be a window and conduit for the other side, but that gift would be of no use if the efficacy of prayer wasn't tapped into. So I prayed, dearly and profusely.

As I was praying, a male soul, slight of frame, with thin, chiseled features and long gray hair, came walking out of the woods. I had no idea who he was. He didn't say a word. He just came up to me and signaled for me to follow him. I was led to a cave, where I sat outside and waited as he disappeared. I had a sense he would come back shortly. I looked at my surroundings and all was still. Then the male spirit reappeared with a number of other male spirits. I didn't recall ever feeling that uncomfortable before, even in ordinary reality. They circled around me, looked at me, and were reticent in their opinions about me. I waited, and slowly, I began to receive information about what happened to some of the Natives and why the souls were having trouble crossing over. I received this information the same way I usually do, through words, pictures, and kinesthetic feelings. Some of the same pictures flashed through my mind: the strife, the famine, the deprivation, the abuse of the women and children, the loss of the land. The medicine healers and spirits of old were continuing their work on the other side, on behalf of those souls who were stuck, and there were more, many more of their people to help. In many religious and spiritual traditions, a living human being whose prayers can reach the heavens is also needed to help with the transition of these stuck souls. There is a biblical reference about when two or more are gathered in his name . . . which can include souls here and in the spirit world.

I was shown some of the tools the medicine men used to use, and some of the games that they would all play as a tribe. I was also given permission by some of the male spirits to work on their land, while the others looked on reluctantly. I thanked them for their trust in me and left.

I went back to where the children and their mothers were playing and sat in the tall grass once again. I drew my rattle up toward the sky and rejoiced, shaking it gently to the beat of the earth I was sitting on.

I looked at a pine tree and wanted to know its medicine. I tuned in to it, moving my hands and feet to become its limbs. I made myself focus strongly on the scent of its needles, so that the aroma could penetrate my being. I hummed whatever melody came out of my mouth and, grabbing my notebook, started to scribble what the pine tree and the spirits of the pine tree were telling me.

Pine medicine . . . helps you find your way when you've lost your sense of direction. Needles were burned to give elders visions. Heals infections of the lungs, throat, ears. Aids in uterine hemorrhaging. Brings the spirit back into the body . . .

One by one, I would touch a tree, tune in to an animal, grab hold of a plant or a flower, touch the earth; whatever I did, I would receive information on the medicinal and spiritual healing qualities of the living things around me.

Prickly ash . . . used in cases of fevers, chills, epidemics. Healed heart troubles, headaches, confusion, hysteria. Brought healing to strife among married partners and relationship issues . . .

White Oak . . . sacred tree, divination tree, has powers of prophecy, protection, clearing of evil spirits, respiratory ailments, male reproductive ailments . . .

Deer, elk, wolf medicine—hours passed as I recorded what I heard, felt, or saw. Whether it was the spirit of a particular thing, or the spirits that protected it, didn't matter.

I was exhausted by nightfall, and when I looked up to see the children and the mothers still playing, it looked as though they were exhausted, too. Something was happening to their spirits, but I hadn't a clue at that time as to what. I gathered myself and wearily walked back to the house. I turned to look behind me as I neared my friends' home because I thought I heard music playing—flute music. I knew there wasn't a soul around for miles; my friends had acquired over a hundred acres of that sacred land, and theirs was the only home on it. I decided I must be hearing things, or that my friends were playing the music.

As I climbed the last hill to the house, the music continued. How lovely, I thought. My friends must have put on a CD and blasted the music at an incredible volume. But when I walked into the house, there was a deadening silence. So much so that I called out to ask if anyone was there. My friend came out of her bedroom and asked me what was wrong. When I asked whether they had been playing any type of flute or Native American music, she looked at me, bewildered, and said no—why? I told her what I'd heard, and she said that it was impossible—there wasn't another home around for miles.

Impossible, or a gift from the spirit world?

I took a long hot shower and went over my notes. I knew my time in the mountains was short, so I wanted to wake up early and get the day started.

At breakfast the next day, my friends asked how my work was going. They also wanted to know if there was anything I could do to improve that parcel of land that was resistant to vegetation growth. I told them I would carry their intentions in my prayers that day.

I went down to my usual spot, which was a ten- or fifteen-minute walk from the house. The spirits started to appear, but a number of the lost children had gone away, as well as a number of the Native children. Hmm . . . perhaps the lost children had helped them cross over. I also saw that some of the women, some of the mothers, had smiles on their faces. Their banter seemed lighter. I was ecstatic. I looked around for the hungry deer; there hardly were any now, as my friends had been leaving food out and the animal spirits had fed upon the food's energies.

I really and truly felt grateful. I was understanding that, in some way, I was giving a voice to the ancients of this land. I was the voice for the trees, the animals, the children, the women. And in giving them a voice as I journaled their stories, I had somehow helped release them, or at the very least initiated that process. That is why the plant remedies in the second half of this book do not just come from one spirit; they come from all the spirits who were involved in the healing work. I might write of only one spirit, elemental, or plant god appearing at any specific time, but it is thanks to all the souls I encountered, from the beginning of this work, that my plant remedies came to be. I continue to know that I am just a vehicle for Spirit.

I sat down on the sun-drenched grass that morning and took out my notebook. At first I stayed on the outskirts of where the women's and children's spirits were playing, but it didn't take me long to get up and move closer. I was smiling; I could feel their laughter. The grass was long and the children's spirits were moving to and fro. The beauty of their auras was something to behold. I moved my body in rhythm to their beat, as though I wanted to join in on their leisurely game. I was in unison. It was lovely.

I played for a while and then sat down again to begin my work. I brought myself into my usual meditative space and asked the spirits of nature and the plant gods to help me gather whatever information I could. In my mind and heart, I was seeing my book come together. The information I was gathering here, the plants I had planted at home . . . all of this would culminate in some sort of story and reference guide.

> The old Indian teaching was that it is wrong to tear loose from its place on the earth anything that may be growing there. It may be cut off, but it should not be uprooted. The trees and the grass have spirits. Whenever one of such growths may be destroyed by some good Indian, his act is done in sadness and with a prayer for forgiveness because of his necessities.
>
> Wooden Leg, Cheyenne

I wanted to understand a bit more about the animal spirits I was seeing. The spirit deer seemed much more at peace. Birds of prey hovered over me in the skies, monitoring my every move. Both in real-world time and in the spirit world, the animals and their spiritual counterparts were joined in harmony, living together naturally. I asked how animal spirit medicine might work in real time. I knew that various cultures have different perspectives, and I wasn't sure if I was even going to receive an answer from those around me.

I took my journal, pen in hand, and waited for the syllables to come into my ears.

Animal spirits give their powers to persons who use their medicine to benefit themselves and their tribal relations. Each of the four-leggeds has a spirit that walks both the earth and the spirit realm. Each spirit has powers given to it by Great Spirit, and by the ancestors who embodied it in times past . . .

The words continued, letting me know that, in their tradition, when someone needed assistance or protection from an animal spirit, he or she could connect to and embody the animal in physical form, energetically and psychically. To gain a deeper understanding of the animal kingdom, the person would attempt to identify with the animal in its entirety, harnessing its powers in order to actually become one with it.

Such identification and connection were useful for traveling the world beyond the earth, below the Spirit, and in any dimension in between. Sometimes the person would take the shape of an animal to retrieve a spirit that was lost or stolen by another. This exchange of form showed all that the two-leggeds were no different from the four-leggeds. All the creatures made by the Great Spirit are one. The more someone practiced this medicine, the more the spirit of the animal and the spirit of the person would become one.

Many times, the animal and its spirit would choose who would carry its energy and, through initiation, strengthen the carrier with more powers. When a warrior could skillfully move from animal to human form, he was unable to be touched or harmed by another. The strength of one man became like that of a thousand.

Animal spirit medicine was also used to help with everyday ritual and ceremony, personal growth, and initiation. Animal spirits acted as guides, protectors, and divination tools, and were called upon when needed. Animals respect the earth and show humans how to embrace it as healers and caretakers. They guide humans in walking gracefully on the earth in the shadows of the powers that be. If you pay close attention to the wisdom that an animal brings you, you can see far into the future and back into the past regarding how your specific relationship with the earth can benefit the present moment—thus influencing both times to come and times past. Do not take an animal or its medicine for granted, for the moment you cease to acknowledge the animal's powers, you disconnect yourself from the source of your energy. Remember, as above, so below. Animal spiritual energies contribute to our earthly existence. Animals, before humans, knew and appreciated the bounty of Mother Earth and revered her energies. It is only because of them and the Creator that we continue to grow and even have a life-form with which to nourish ourselves. Think about it.

Fusing with an animal's energy was one of the ways in which a person could understand the created world and its Creator, and also the relationships between the animal kingdom and other kingdoms. Once people felt they could conquer the animal kingdom, however, they often felt they could conquer all others, which led them to abandon the respect we owe to the four-leggeds and to the Creator. As human beings, we have to be very watchful of our need for power and respect the laws of nature as granted from above. Identifying with an animal can also help us understand our role and relationship to power, as given to us by the Creator. There was once a time when humans and animals shared their powers collectively in nature, and when reverence for the Creator was shared evenly.

Present day animals have become wary because humans fail to recognize them as an important and necessary part of their own creation. Men and women derive their instinctual practices and behaviors from animals, and sexual instincts originally derive from the energies of the animal kingdom. Then they evolve, rising up toward the Creator through the plant kingdom, seeking the higher energies of the Divine. Humans often confuse their relationship to themselves as sexual beings with their primal instincts and cease to acknowledge a higher sexual aspiration toward the heavens. The primal instincts of the animal kingdom, however, are in fact meant to lead to the awareness of the magic of creation—through the energies that the plant kingdom offers. It is the shared process of awakening, of moving from birth to death, that connects the animal kingdom to the plant kingdom. It is how the story of creation gives rise to the powers and manifestations of the Creator. It is how all things connect and open to the heavens.

> We know ourselves to be made of this earth.
> We know this earth is made from our bodies.
> For we see ourselves. And we are nature.
> We are nature seeing nature.
>
> *Susan Griffin*

The animal spirit is meant to bridge the world so that humans can enter into alternate realities. It differs from the plant spirit in its intention and essence. Whether or not a traveler knows this, every human is protected by some form of spiritual energy that embraces nature. But sometimes people refuse to utilize all their resources when aspiring to the heavens through the natural world.

Animal spirit medicine can also give you knowledge of the plant kingdom. The four-leggeds of the earth were the first to utilize plant spirit medicine and gave it freely to humans with the understanding that their use of the natural world would be in right relationship to the heavens. When this did not occur, human relationships with both the animal and the plant kingdoms suffered. People now need to once again earn the trust of the natural world.

You cannot honor one kingdom without honoring all.

As the words stopped coming, a butterfly fluttered at the ends of my long hair as they whispered in the gentle breeze. I acknowledged the spirits and gave thanks for the voices and their words. I felt like I had connected more deeply with the spirits of the deer; it seemed there had been a purpose for their suffering.

I got up to stretch my legs and take a brief stroll. I wanted to walk to the barren vegetable garden that my friends were concerned about. But there was nothing remarkable about it when I arrived there; it simply looked like dirt in an unplowed field, parched from drought even though everything else around it was lush. It was about one-fifth of an acre of land. The sun was still shining in splendor on every blade of grass, every tree branch, and every flower around me. Even this desolate piece of land glowed, with the sun's warming rays upon it.

I decided to sit in the middle of the parcel and do some of my work there. My intentions were that I would eventually find out what had happened there. As I lay down my satchel and tools, I became very hot and my body started to itch. I just let it pass through me and focused on the next flower or tree—whatever it was that spirit wanted me to work with. And so I began, one by one, to work with whomever wanted to lend their voice to me.

> *Red chestnut medicine . . . used to assist women going through the change of life. Drinking the tea made out of bark used for hysteria. It would call the spirit of the mind back home. Used for miscarriages and for protecting the mother from malevolent spirits when she was grieving for her child . . .*
>
> *Beech medicine . . . used as a blood purifier, for rheumatism and for tuberculosis. Helps with protection in childhood against physical deformity. Paste of the bark used for broken limbs. Paste also healed wounds. Treated childhood vascular ailments . . .*
>
> *Mulberry Bush . . . used to dispel poisons; acts as an emetic. When planted outside of a home, keeps away all unwanted critters. A paste of the berries helps with poison ivy and other skin rashes . . .*

I took a break for a moment, looking up from my writing to get a breath of fresh air. My hands were so hot from writing, and I'd temporarily stopped noticing the physical sensations I'd experienced when I first sat down. To my surprise, I saw my shaman, standing there and watching with pride as I did my work. I also saw the male spirit I'd met the other day, the one who took me to that cave, as well as a few of the other male spirits who had been there. The women's and children's spirits were also not far from me, and elementals and devas and other spirits of nature abounded. We all seemed to be in one harmonious interplay. I felt peaceful when seeing those around me so peaceful. It left an ineffable feeling in my heart.

After a long moment, I turned back to my writing. The rush of heat that went through my body again spurred my hand to start taking down notes and caused syllables to begin echoing in my ears. The words came and I became one with them.

Medicine of plant spirits . . . in working with the aforementioned, it is not about the curative practice of the plant medicine itself or even its connection with the elemental. Without our commitment to bringing balance to the consciousness of humans in regard to caretaking of the earth, the medicine means nothing to the spirit or the plant god who offers it to you. It is they who need us to take responsibility for the healing of the earth's peoples, its creatures, and its land throughout all time. We are the gatekeepers and if the earth continues to die, then we are responsible for the death of its spirit and all those spirits who reside within its many spiritual dimensions . . .

What I'd just written sent chills down my spine. It is true that when I first began doing this work and would take a leaf from a flowering plant or a piece of branch from a tree to retrieve its medicine, I noticed that after I was finished hearing its voice, the spiritual energy of the living thing in my hand was totally gone. But please know that whenever I took a part of a tree or flower, I asked permission first. Many times, of course, I just tuned in to the flower or tree in order to be its voice.

I felt that I wanted to know more about children—children of the past, the present, and the future. Since they had been around me for a while in my own spiritual process, I was hoping to have some understanding in their role, as understood by the energies around me. The words came:

Children are a sign of both the past and things to come. Anyone who has placed black magic on a child will fall prey to his own making. It was said that when children were born ill, they had taken it upon themselves in agreement with the Great Spirit to carry the ills of the earth, its caretakers, and the ancestors before them. Some of those specially gifted children will be the great peacemakers of times to come.

Karma carries itself heavily on the little ones, and what would be their greatest weakness will be their greatest strength as they get older, if they chose to utilize the gifts that were given to them in the midst of their suffering.

It is very easy for children to lose sight of their spirits and give them over to another, as there will be many who prey on the spirits of young ones. There is sometimes fear and confusion left over from the ancestral energies of another soul, which then embodies itself in the young one. It is up to the elders of any time continuum to retrieve the spirit of the young child back from wherever it has departed and to send away the ancestral energy. It is the responsibility of every elder to watch over a child, whether or not it belongs to him . . .

I laughed for a moment in recognition. There's a bumper sticker I always love to see on the back of cars: "It takes a village to raise a child." The voice I was hearing through the ethers was saying the same.

I looked up, and oddly enough, it seemed as though some of the women's and children's souls had disappeared. I wasn't worried, because all the other protective souls were still around me. I assumed the women and children had crossed while I was writing. No, I was sure of it.

I wrote for a little while longer and was growing tired. I ate some of my bag lunch and hoped that with renewed strength and vigor, I would be able to figure out the cause of the land's bareness and glean whether any vegetation could grow on it in the future.

I lay down for a while and let the sun's moist heat brown my arms and my face. Ever since childhood, I've loved the feeling of lying on the earth. That and snowflakes falling are my two fondest nature memories. I always felt so secure, so protected in these magical energies.

The heat on my face shifted. When I opened my eyes, I saw that the clouds had moved and now blocked the sunlight. That was a sign for me to get up and tune in to the land, as much as the spirits would allow. I took a deep breath and prayed. The physical sensations I'd felt earlier started to reappear. Intense heat and itching were dominant. I allowed these energies to expand so that I could be clearer about them. As I did, I remembered to call upon every voice of that land that had given me access to its light, and every plant spirit that I had been introduced to thus far. I realized why my shaman was there—to give me extra protection.

> I am you and you are me; wherever you are, I am there. And I am scattered in all things; from wherever you want to, you gather Me; and in gathering Me, you gather yourself.
>
> *Gospel of Eve*

As the energies moved through me, I couldn't breathe. It felt as though my lungs were filling up with smoke and it became dark around me. I could hear screams and cries, and the earth felt like it was moving under me. Animals were scattering in confusion and disarray as I was somehow energetically being transported back to another time. The visions started to come, and I could see glimpses of the massacre that had taken place.

I had previously known that there was bloodshed in this land, but there was something unique about this particular piece of land. It was here, I realized, that the women and children had been taken and raped, abused, separated, and tortured. The women and children I now saw seemed to number in the hundreds—new faces, more than I had been allowed to observe before. The fires, many of them, and the flames were constant . . . it was a continual burning. All the people were suffering. At that time, it was not unusual for male warriors or tribesmen to be killed in a massacre, but for this number of women's lives to be taken was in some way abominable. And for some reason, their souls took hold of the land . . . so that if they became lost in the spirit world, they could find each other here.

I somehow understood that. This land had acted as a womb to these women, the seat of power where life and death begins and ends. One of the connections they had to the earth and to what was transpiring was this piece of ground I was sitting on. How could anything grow on it now? Its soul had been taken away. The grief I felt around me was profound, and part of what the spirits wanted was recognition. But these visions and feelings were more than I'd wanted to experience. I brought myself out of my meditative space and got up quickly. I was done for the day.

I went back to the house and my friends. I told them about my visions, and they asked if there was anything they could do. My answer will always be the same to anyone who asks that question: *pray*. Simply, undeniably, inexorably pray.

I went to bed and asked for a medicine dream. Was there anything that the spirits needed me to do in my prayers, to repent for what had happened? If so, I would be open to it. Not that I thought what transpired was my fault in any way, but on an energetic level we all need to share the responsibility, just as I heard the voices tell me.

My sleep was erratic. I tossed and turned until the early hours of the morning. I had a glass of water by my bed, but it wasn't enough to quench my thirst. Lines of sweat rolled down my forehead. It felt like I was still attached to the heat I'd felt on the land—heat that was partially from those fires burning—and I would think of the cumulative anger that arose about the atrocities taking place. I was itchy again and did what I could to fall asleep. Somehow I managed to, because the next thing I knew I was dreaming.

In my dreams, I saw a gathering of Native American women dancing around a fire. There was one in particular that I noticed; she was short in stature but full-bodied. The lines of her face were drawn with character, matching her strength, wisdom, and maturity. I knew she was a healer, a medicine woman, a person of peace. She was leading the others in a tribal dance and motioning me to come and join in. She chanted, and then moved her body upward toward the sky, and then downward toward the earth, allowing her entire being to touch and merge with the earth. She offered herself and the soul of her womb to the Great Mother, cradling the ground as she searched for a peaceful energy that would come forth. As she sprang upward, branches of black cohosh appeared in her hand. She danced around the fire, touching every woman with it. She also came over to me and blessed me with it. I stayed back from the fire and the other women in my dream, since I felt uncomfortable. She spoke in a language that I couldn't understand, but the words of her prayer I heard clearly.

O sacred grounds of the earth, lull our spirits to rest upon your divine heartbeat. Take from us our pain so that you may transform it with your profound healing energy.

They all danced that prayer, their faces entranced by the sacredness of the chant and their medicine woman. The fire glowed radiantly as, one by one, they seemed to draw near to it to give it thanks. In my mind, I asked the medicine woman if there was any way I could make an offering to the souls who had perished on that land, and to the physical land itself. I had a feeling she knew that my friends wanted to grow vegetation on it, but she did not address that issue. She showed me, through her eyes, that I should gather myself and my friends on that land and to do a ceremony. She wanted a black cohosh planted in the middle of that land with some stones around it—a sort of sanctuary. She asked for lots of prayers and let me know that all would be present.

I woke up the next day a little excited. I ran to breakfast and told my friends to retrieve a black cohosh plant and call a few other friends up. In the afternoon, a few of us went down to the site, including a friend who facilitated sweat lodges. We all gathered in a circle and called in the spirits. We'd brought offerings, which we placed in the middle of the one-fifth acre of land along with the black cohosh. One by one, we offered prayers out loud. After the last person spoke, I went into a deeper space, allowing the visions and feelings to come once more so that we might all become one with them. I remembered the plant spirit prayer of the black cohosh and said it aloud so that one and all could hear.

> *O sacred grounds of the earth, lull our spirits to rest upon your divine heartbeat. Take from us our pain so that you may transform it with your profound healing energy.*

I repeated the words numerous times and began to feel the heat rise up in my body and the itching start. The visions and physical sensations were coming more quickly this time. I recounted them aloud, so that everyone would know what I saw and heard.

The blaze of the fires seemed greater in this vision. The children's cries went through my bones. There was one little one, with scorch marks on his face, running with outstretched hands and screaming for his mother. He found her. There were grandmothers and grandfathers, too old and feeble to walk fast enough to escape the flames that seemed to engulf them from every direction. They did what they could to help their adult children and the little ones. The elders couldn't fight off the enemies who would torture the women and hurt the children—there were just too many of them. They tried. They fought valiantly as lives were taken. I kept looking around to find the able-bodied men of the clan, but they were few and far between. Whether they were away at war themselves or on a hunt I did not know. All I saw was the lack of protection that these souls had.

I repeated these visions over and over, along with whatever else came to me. I started to sound verbose, but I just couldn't fathom what I was seeing. When I intermittently brought myself out of the visions,

I could see the astonished and guilty looks on my friends' faces. What did they have to feel guilty about? Perhaps their compassion led them to feel universally responsible, as it did for me, and it was clear by the looks on their faces that they wanted to do something. They all were starting to feel physical sensations as I talked. I kept talking until the energies—of the visions we were seeing and of the thoughts and emotions that united us as one—went through me. I could see my shaman in the ethers, holding the space for all of us.

After twenty minutes or so, the visions subsided, as did the physical feelings and emotions that we were all experiencing. We threw some tobacco on the ground, along with whatever else we brought that was holy. We adorned the black cohosh with some more natural decorations and offered our sanctuary up to the souls who were lost. It didn't seem important anymore to my friends that this land yield a harvest. The air had become cold, and we closed the space and left the spirits in peace.

I had one more day left in the mountains. I finished up my work and felt sad about leaving. I wanted to get back home, though, to attend to the plants I'd planted for my book, and I also missed my cats. The day went by quickly, and the next thing I knew my bags were packed and already in the van for the train station.

We were running late, but I wanted to say a quick goodbye to my friends of the mountains, forest, and sacred land. They knew I was coming—the spirits, I mean. I went to my usual place and hundreds of souls walked out among the trees. It really was an image to behold. They were luminous. No words were spoken, but feelings were exchanged from heart to heart. I did hear one message, though. They asked me to look down right where I was standing, because there was a present for me. Not even half a foot away from my feet was a feather. I picked up the feather and said thank-you.

I waved goodbye and told them I would miss them. I ran back to the house; my friends were waiting in the van for me. I showed them the feather. One of my friends, an avid bird watcher, said it was impossible that that feather would be found in this part of the country. The bird it belonged to wasn't indigenous to the area, or even to anywhere nearby. Unfortunately, I can't recall the name of the bird. And maybe we were mistaken . . .

An hour into the drive to the train station, we turned on the radio and were listening to an announcer talk about the mundane. Then, in the course of his banter, he mentioned this bird out of the blue and talked about the significance of it. My friends and I just looked at one another, and the confounded looks on our faces was enough of a confirmation that the feather was truly a gift to me from the spirit world.

I keep the feather on one of my bookshelves, framed. And oh yes—a year after our ceremony, vegetation started to grow on that barren area of my friends' land.

I arrived back home after a twenty-hour ordeal on the train. I love the scenic route of the railroad . . . I just didn't realize how tiring it would all be.

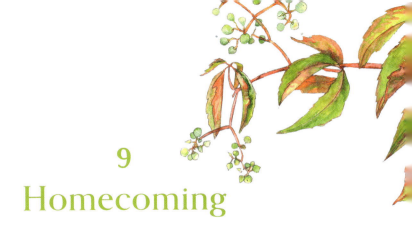

9
Homecoming

The first thing I wanted to do when I walked in the house was to see my cats. Ceara came up to me and greeted me as usual, and when I looked for Alexis, I spotted her in the corner. I went over to her where she huddled but she pulled away from my touch. I looked closer and saw that she had a six-inch African porcupine quill sticking out of her neck. After I called my mother in a panic, I rushed Alexis to the vet. She was incredibly lucky, but the vet kept asking me why my cat had a porcupine quill stuck in her neck. He said that the way it was jammed in, it looked as though someone had stabbed her with it.

That needle had been lying atop one of my shelves, out of sight. There was no way Alexis could get to it. I know that sometimes in our work, even though we are protected and taught to stay in the light, there are malevolent spirits who do harm. I felt that this was what happened to Alexis. During my most recent work with the plants, I had seen how animals take on our issues and protect us from harm. As I left the vet's office and took Alexis home, I saw the spirits who protected her—the Native Americans and the animal spirits and, of course, the plants. It was pretty miraculous.

I took a break for a few weeks, tending to clients and checking in on my garden. I had a lot of material already for my book and soon would gather the plants and give them a voice too. My shaman was around again, more so than ever. It felt good to be back. Over the past few months with my clients, I'd utilized what I'd learned in a more conscious way; although I'd been working along these lines to some degree all along, the effectiveness and privileges bestowed by those above and beyond are tenfold after they initiate you into their medicine and healing world.

Two weeks seemed more than enough time to rest, as far as my shaman was concerned. It was time to start gathering plants. I began to perceive that I would also make medicines, flower essences, and plant spirit remedies. A friend of mine who owned an herbal apothecary taught me how to make the medicines, and when I was working with them, the process was refined by nature and the elementals.

> When you care for one tree, all the trees smile.
> *Laura Silvana Aversano*

It was a Monday when I gathered the first leaf from the first plant that I wanted to voice. I didn't feel the need to always work with the flowers if they were in bloom; I wanted to touch the green. I wanted to feel the plant's extremities. I went into my small urban backyard on a very rainy day and just stopped at the first plant that was calling me. Calendula. *Calendula officinalis*. The flowers were indeed in bloom. I took one of them, but I decided I would work with a leaf as well. As always, I asked permission from the plant and its protectors and then put down a small gift. Sometimes I give something sweet. The earth and its spiritual inhabitants really do have a sweet tooth!

I took the calendula flower and leaf inside and went into my living room. My candles were lit, and I think both of the cats were hanging out (they always loved being a part of my work; Ceara would come to sessions and Alexis would quietly assist me in her own way). I sat down on my red carpet and held the calendula in my hand, with my journal and pen sitting in front of me.

Just as my shaman had taught me, I tuned in to calendula and waited for its prayer.

Play with me, O joyful one, and shine your radiance under the sun. Bring comfort, joy, and innocence to all, for we behold your beauty for one so small.

I paused, then burst into prayer, feeling a beatific smile come across my face.

Play with me, O joyful one, and shine your radiance under the sun. Bring comfort, joy, and innocence to all, for we behold your beauty for one so small.

The little leaf was vibrating in my hand. My living room turned into a magical place each time I worked with a plant to channel its healing energies and medicine. It would become misty from the ethers and from the spirits who formed around me. I waited for the calendula elemental to appear. I knew my shaman was with me. Actually, a few plant gods were present. I had made many friends on my trip to the mountains and found that I had acquired new teachers in the spirit world—new medicine men and women and new plant gods—to assist me in my work. They didn't belong to me; I was still their child, wanting to learn whatever it is they wanted to teach me. My shaman and I were close—he felt more like family to me. As a child I had always loved school and wanted to become close with my teachers; it was the same now that I was an adult, only these teachers were beyond the veil. I hungered for knowledge and for their approval and hoped that I was disciplined enough to earn whatever gems of wisdom they might bestow on me.

They were all present this day to watch me learn from the plants and their elementals. They would not interfere unless I was headed down the wrong path. I had a sense that some of them might even have been proud of me.

I called to calendula. Excitedly, a little girl appeared to me. She was surrounded by butterflies and flowers, and all of God's creatures abounded. My living room was Paradise in an instant. She was joyful. Growing near to her was an abundant amount of calendula. She became smitten with its flowers, and the magic enticed her to dance upon its soft earthen petals. Birds fluttered through the strands of yellow hair that flew from her small head. She was drunk with calendula's healing magic and made a sacred pact, the kind that only children can make, with the calendula plant. She wanted to share its medicine with every living creature under the sun.

I relished this vision for a few moments, and then my writing hand became inflamed with heat. I knew it was time to pick up my pen and journal.

> *The spirit of this plant is called upon to help children . . . it helps them feel safe in a world where they might be alone . . . heals the inner child . . . reconnects one with their lost innocence . . . brings laughter, creates boundaries . . . tonifies the thymus gland, improves cognitive function, alleviates muscle tension . . . an herbal oil infused with calendula is good for joint pain . . .*

My hand went on and on and on. I think I wrote about calendula for an hour. Then again, all of the plants took me at least that long. As each emotion passed through me, I would feel each physical ailment in my tissues, organs, muscles, and bones.

I hadn't realized it, but by the time I was finished with calendula, the leaf had withered to such an extent in my palm that it had started to fall apart. I remembered something similar happening on my trip to the mountains. I was tired after each session with a plant, but my body and mind were clearer. While the flora in the mountains belonged to the mountains, the energy was a little different with the plants I'd grown in my backyard. They had been cultivated with New York City energy and with my hard work, love, and attention. My connection with them felt more personal.

I worked with two plants each day. Some of their elementals were a little too eager to become my friends. I remember once, at about four in the morning, I was woken from a deep sleep by the spirit of dandelion flying through my room. I was saddened over the loss of a close friend and had been grieving since the week before. I woke up because someone was tickling me. Thinking I was dreaming, I went back to sleep then was woken up again. I saw a young boy whizzing like a fairy across my bedroom, laughing gleefully and trying to play with me. I don't think he cared what time it was; he just wanted to make me smile!

Strange things were happening those weeks that I worked with the plants. My physical body remained strong, but funny things were happening around me and I knew it had to do with the plants. I would misplace things, things kept dropping, the cats were scattered. Nothing that occurred felt negative; it all just seemed so haphazard.

Dandelion was a very fun plant to work with. The morning I went into my backyard to gather its flower and leaf, I saw a stray cat who was staying around the garden throughout this time. He protected the garden, and he seemed to be protective of me. He would wait for me on my front stoop when I went out at night, and when I came home, he waited for me to go through my front door and then left. (I named him Sammie; after I finished my work with the plants, Sammie found a loving home with my mom and her dog. He is still happily enjoying himself in her abode with her other pets and of course, my mom's array of houseplants.) Sammie watched placidly as I tiptoed between the plants, seeking out the dandelion. It was actually a bit hard to find because it was also growing all over my backyard and in the little patch of soil in front of my house. But I wanted to procure the flower and leaf from the specific plant I'd been praying over ever since I planted it.

The golden-yellow petals of its flower were so astounding that I didn't want to injure the plant at all. I bent down to it and gently placed my fingers around the stem, asking permission to take a flower and a leaf. When I felt I'd been given the go-ahead to do so, I gracefully plucked the flower and leaf. With these two living things in my hand, I went back into my living room and sat on the floor once again. Once I started to pray, it didn't take long for the mist to appear. Candles were lit, and all that I needed was placed on the floor in front of me.

Joyful spirit, full of glee, fill me, embrace me, and shelter me. Make this magic of the most high, grant my dreams unto the sky.

It didn't take long for that whimsical young boy with the fairylike energy to come flying by me. I don't think I'd even uttered the last word of the prayer. Wherever he flew, a rainbow trailed behind him. I could tell he loved rainbows because he would look behind him after each one appeared and smile. The colors in this vision were so real that I could touch them. Even this young magical boy exuded colors—he emoted colors. When he smiled, brilliant colors appeared in his aura. He was very empathic, so if he picked up on an emotion from me, various colors appeared. That was one of his gifts. He so loved the golden-yellow hues of dandelion. He sat atop some of his rainbows and showed me that he could grant wishes to people in honor of the dandelion.

The energy of the vision was halted by my hand heating up again. I began to write whatever came through.

Helps with depression and sadness . . . assists with grief and loss . . . gives strength during a soul loss, deals with shock, sudden trauma, loss . . . brings abundance and good fortune . . .

Good remedy for headaches and sinus infections . . . mucus in the lungs, lowers blood pressure, increases circulation, energy surrounding diabetes . . .

I wrote until the words stopped flowing, and as with all the other plants whose energy was channeled through me, the emotions and the physical ailments became part of me for a few moments in time. At the end of the session, as I expected, the flower and the leaf had given their life-force and withered.

I spent a few days doing this each week until I was done with the thirty plants that I'd grown in my garden. My book was coming together. I hadn't yet put anything formal into a computer—all my notes were written with pen on paper—but I was elated.

Still to come, however, were the flower essences, or remedies. Having just finished working with the plants themselves, I couldn't wait to make my thirty mother tinctures. (Mother tinctures are the first stage of a vibrational remedy, incorporating a plant, animal, or mineral substance in a mixture of water and alcohol.) I had originally intended to take a break and wait a few weeks before starting this process; I wanted to focus on my clients and invite the new spiritual energies I'd been working with into my practice. But one evening on the local news, they announced that the spraying would soon begin again. I was very angry, to say the least. The powers that be were all concerned about the West Nile virus, yet the pesticides were what posed the greater risk.

Previously, I had called my local councilman and put in a civilian complaint letting them know that I'd gotten sick from the spraying. They said they'd never heard of such a thing; but, of course, the first time a neurotoxin was sprayed, there were so many news reports of people having reactions from it that they changed the pesticide the following year. I was concerned once again—it had taken me a while to rebalance myself and I didn't want to go through that again. I decided to take the necessary precautions and just do what I could. That also meant I had to harvest the leaves from the plants to make the remedies earlier than planned.

It rained for a few days. I hoped the rain would continue, since it would put off the aerial spraying. It soaked the ground and the plants seemed to skyrocket. At my living room table, I prepared a number of crystal glasses that had been handed down from my Italian grandmother. I filled them with water and labeled them with their respective plant names. I had the other materials in place to make the remedies: I'd ordered the tincture bottles weeks beforehand, and I'd collected a few plant leaves at a time. I used very few blossoms for the mother tinctures—I was called to mostly use the leaves. I placed the leaves, one by one, in their coordinating crystal glasses, and when all of the thirty plants were floating atop the water in each glass, the work of making the remedy begun.

I prayed, I chanted. I used all the plant spirit prayers that had been given to me by the spirits and elementals of the natural world. I lit candles and let the glow of the candlelight surround them. The next day was supposed to be bright and sunny, so I was hoping to leave them overnight, embraced by the gentle energies of the heavens, and then place them in the early morning sunlight to be blessed.

I couldn't have asked for a better day when I woke up. Still in my pajamas, I ran into the living room, retrieved the crystal glasses two at a time, and went into my garden to place them in the walkway. Sammie, my outdoor stray, was watching as usual. My intention was to leave the glasses in the sunlight for an hour and then begin to make and bottle the tinctures. I sat next to Sammie as all the glasses glistened in the sunlight. The leaves, interestingly enough, were not withered; they still had life to them. And I could tell that the energy of the water inside each glass was different. I prayed and asked all of nature to bless these remedies. When the time came, I made each tincture with such gratitude for the medicine I was honored to work with.

> I cured with the power that came through me.
> Of course, it was not I who cured, it was the power
> from the outer world. The visions and the ceremonies
> had only made me like a hole through which the power

> could come to the two-leggeds. If I thought
> I was doing it myself, the hole would close up
> and no power could come through. Then everything
> I could do would be foolish.
>
> *Black Elk*

So much had happened over the last few months. I tried to piece together my destiny, as it were—the miasm, my mother's gifts, my gifts. My mom always said that before I was born, she was told she was going to have a daughter who would write books and help people. I had lived a lifetime in the past year, and putting my book together would be my way of honoring not only the spirits and their teachings, but my family ancestry.

I settled in, in preparation for the chemical spraying that would start in a few days. I felt that I was more physically prepared than last time and stronger on all levels. And with what felt like most of the miasm cleared, I hoped I would respond differently to the pesticides. But I didn't expect what happened next.

It was an excruciatingly hot day when the helicopters hovered and released their poisons. I closed all the windows, shut off the air conditioner, and planned not to leave the house until hours after it was over. The local department of environmental protection actually recommended that anyone with allergies or who was immunosuppressed stay indoors.

I had lots of work to do, so that wasn't an issue. The spraying started early in the morning, but it wasn't until dusk that they came to spray the areas close to me. I live near the water, and when there is a gentle breeze, you can feel and smell the pesticides intensify as they come your way.

The day passed and I distracted myself. I wanted it to be just another day; I stayed positive about any reaction I might have. Evening came. I cooked dinner and kept myself occupied until bedtime. Morning arrived, and I felt secure enough to venture out into the neighborhood and take care of some errands before my work started. My sense of smell is so sensitive that I could indeed smell the toxins as I walked out of my house. (Friends told me their allergies were heightened, and sensitive clients had reacted to the pesticide as well.) Over the next few days, I started getting headaches and my face took on a yellowish color, and I knew that my thyroid was affected once again. The effects weren't as intense as with the last round of spraying, but I still did not want to have to deal with them.

I'd heard about an urban shaman who practiced fifteen minutes away from me. I had never gone to her before but decided to give something different a try. I called for an appointment and got one rather quickly. I felt a bit like we were kindred spirits when we met. I could hear the spirits talking over her, suggesting remedies for me—one of them was for detoxing and one of them was for spiritual protection. She said I needed both. But I was disoriented that day due to the headache and light-headedness, and I didn't correctly write down everything she told me to do. She was from one of the islands in the Caribbean, and the herbs she suggested were indigenous to that region, so I wasn't acquainted with them.

I left my appointment feeling reassured that along with my continued methods of healing, the medicinals and suggestions this urban shaman made would clear me of this pesticide residue once and for all. After this spraying, I had a sense that my reactions each time would be lessened. I would turn out to be right.

I waited a few days before starting the remedies. The effects of the sprays were continuing to work their way through my body, and I paid close attention to eating the right foods and cleansing. My sleep patterns were very much changed, and my senses were extremely heightened. I felt, once again, more "open" than usual and didn't want to be in large crowds. I also found myself reacting to things I had never reacted to before. This was something new and didn't occur with the last round of spraying. I became sensitive to foods that I'd tolerated previously;

lotions, creams, and even things made with the purest of ingredients made my body feel uncomfortable. I was having what felt like an all-over allergy response. The usual burning and swelling up of various parts of my body occurred, and I was getting frustrated at the thought of this happening all over again.

I finally started using the two remedies the shaman had given me, setting aside things I was already taking so that I could feel the effects of these medicinals alone. I made a tea out of both herbs. I was to drink two cups a day of the one she'd given me to detox my body. The other was from a bush, and she'd given me a pound of the roots. It was used in her native home to protect oneself from malevolent spirits. When we'd met, however, I'd grossly misunderstood her and thought she'd suggested that I drink five to eight cups a day of this root. What she actually suggested was that I take five to eight sips throughout the day, since this is a toxic substance if taken in higher doses. I drank five cups that first day!

Well, after the first few cups, I was so energized that I wanted to know all I could about the herb I was taking. I couldn't find anything, given the slang name the shaman had given me. I trusted her and figured I would come across it within the next few days, so I wasn't concerned. My body was feeling stronger, so I thought it was working.

I continued to drink, and over the next three days upped the dosage by a cup or two. By day three I was so euphoric that I wasn't sleeping at all. I'd visited my acupuncturist for a session, and he'd remarked that he'd never seen my pulses like that. He said they didn't feel like my pulses and that they were all pretty good. He was curious about what I was taking, but he wasn't himself familiar with the plant.

I went home and figured all was good. By day four, I noticed that my cat Alexis was sleeping on me, specifically on my abdomen right over my liver. My high had ended, and over the next few days I lowered the dosage for some reason and started to crash. I needed to rest in between work and each time, Alexis would sit on top of me and sleep on my liver. By day six, I had stopped taking the medicinal and went online to find this plant. By the grace of God, I came upon it and saw that it was in the same family as mistletoe. My mouth dropped open, since I knew how toxic this herb was, and I called the urban shaman immediately. When I told her how much I had been consuming, she gasped and said she had never heard of anyone even able to consume that much without serious harm being done.

I made an appointment the next day with my internist and told him what had happened. He just looked at me, stunned, and did all the necessary tests to make sure I didn't have liver damage and that my heart was functioning normally. He took some blood for testing, and to our surprise, I was not affected at all by the overdose. Everyone who knew what had transpired was amazed. I was just grateful and felt so stupid that I had misheard the instructions.

I spent the next month detoxing from both the medicinal and the pesticide. Even though it was a toxic dose, it had seemed to do the trick. My cleansing was pretty cathartic, and my body became stronger than it had been before, and the pesticides came out faster than they had in the last round of spraying. Each night, Alexis would sleep on me in the same area, giving me comfort as my body burned and sweated out the poisons.

Time went by, and I knew things were clearing up. Alexis also went back to her usual sleeping space on one of the many pillows next to me. I remember thinking one day that she looked great because she had gained a little weight, but then the weight kept coming and I knew something wasn't right.

I made an appointment with my vet. I wasn't concerned and thought maybe her thyroid was out of balance. She'd helped me through my cleansing, and for sure it had affected her somehow. When the vet came in to examine her, he saw her stomach distended and wanted to get some X-rays. It was at that point that I said to myself, "Alexis has liver cancer." The vet came back into the room after about a half hour and told me the news. Most likely it was cancer, but it needed to be confirmed with an ultrasound.

Words cannot express what was going through my mind. The vet drained the fluids out of Alexis's abdomen to make her more comfortable, and we came back a few days later for the ultrasound. My fears were confirmed and Alexis was diagnosed with hepatic cancer. The vet said her prognosis was grim and that surgery would not be useful in this case, nor chemotherapy. The fluids would continuously build up in her abdomen and then possibly her lungs, causing suffocation. They needed to be drained every few days, so I asked the vet to show me how. I did this with Alexis at home.

I brought Alexis back home from that appointment and just looked at her. That was why she had been lying on my liver all those nights. That was why my tests had come out okay. She'd taken the side effects of the medicinals from me. Was it supposed to happen like this? With all the work I'd just done with the plant elementals and the plant gods, weren't they going to save her?

I was angry. I was angry with the spirit world, with God, with myself, with the shaman. I was angry at everyone and everything. I was in shock and couldn't accept that within a month or so, I would lose something so precious to me.

I stayed up late that night. I took out my rosary and prayed really hard. When I finished with my novenas, I prayed to the plant gods. Then I prayed to the elementals. I prayed and asked every spirit that I'd met over the past year to save the life of my cat.

The days went by slowly during her decline. Alexis was able to walk and eat and play for those first two weeks after her diagnosis, so I thought maybe she could be cured. Every day I called upon a different plant, one that had grown in the garden. I called upon black cohosh and feverfew. I prayed to motherwort and blessed thistle. I chanted the prayers to clematis and violet. And one by one, they all came and surrounded her. I remember clearly the day Alexis was sitting on my sofa and I saw the Native American spirits talking to her. Her ears were pointed upward as if she was listening. I still thought for sure a miracle would happen. How could it not, with all these spirits coming to help her?

By the third week, Alexis grew weak and weary. She wasn't able to walk well, so I would bring food to where she lay. She couldn't jump up on the bed to sleep with me, so I put up steps for her to climb. I started to think that a miracle wasn't going to happen, that the spirits didn't listen to my prayers. She started having pain in her right front paw and she would stick her paw into her drinking bowl to cool it off. I kept asking her if it was time for her to go and if so, it would be okay. If she needed assistance, she should just let me know. But she was a fighter and I realized that the time was near, but not yet.

Over a weekend, the signs became clearer. Alexis stopped coming near me and slept in the living room. She lost most of her appetite and was nursing the paw that hurt her. Spirits that I hadn't seen in a while started to appear. My shaman was constantly around and loved Alexis. John, the soul from the cemetery, was around. The lost children were around. And some of the spirits I had befriended from my trip to the mountains were around. I didn't have the emotional energy to tune in to why they were there, since I was so despondent over Alexis. The house was becoming cold, despite the warmth of the energy those spirits brought. Eventually, I couldn't ignore them any longer and wanted to understand why they were here. I knew Alexis had taken on my stuff. Were there other reasons that this had happened?

Apparently there were. The residual energies of the miasm needed to complete themselves. Sometimes, when an ancestral pattern is this big and has a lot of karma attached to it, there is a die-off reaction, so to speak. Something in physical form has to return to where it came from. It doesn't always mean a physical death, but there is a death on many levels that has to occur for completion—and sometimes, unfortunately, in the physical realm as well. Alexis had lovingly offered to assist me with bringing this miasm to completion. She took on the residuals of the pesticides and the medicinals that were lodged in my liver and lymph glands, as well as the energy of the many spirits that were still stuck in my energy field and needed to cross over. They couldn't cross until something else was sacrificed and another piece of spiritual work was complete. There were some of the lost children who were frightened to cross over, and the soul of a beloved pet seemed to comfort their fears.

Alexis also held on to things that I had been carrying for the last fifteen years, and it was time for her to let them go. It was time for my body to be given a different boundary with these ancestors and to purge some of their weaknesses. Alexis knew that. I wasn't ready for her to go, but she knew it was time. John, the soul from the cemetery, came to bring me comfort and support and to assure me that Alexis would be okay. In fact, it seemed as if all the spirits who were present knew of this beforehand; it seemed like they were all waiting for her. I was continually reassured that Alexis would be okay with her transition and that she would be able to see me and her sister Ceara when she crossed. She would be able to visit and play any time she wanted.

It seemed as if I had no choice. There was no bargaining here, and destiny was at play. All were eagerly waiting for her to cross.

The day came, and Alexis cried a cry that I had never heard. She looked at me to say goodbye, but she had trouble dying. I told her it would be okay and brought her to the vet to be euthanized. We had had animals all our lives growing up, but I had never been with one when we had to put them to sleep.

That night was one of the saddest I could remember in a long time. I had lost an animal companion. More than that—she had saved my life, even more than I realized. When I came home from the vet and walked into my living room, I saw all the spirits dancing. I wasn't happy, so I obviously didn't join in. I sat on my bed crying and felt a cat jump on the bed behind me. I thought it was Ceara coming to comfort me but when I turned around, I saw indentations going onto the pillow near where I put my head to sleep—and no physical cat there. I stared in disbelief. At that moment, Ceara jumped onto the bed and sat next to me. We both just stared at the pillow without moving. We knew Alexis was with us, lying on her pillow. All was well.

I slept that night. I slept long and hard. When I awoke, life was different. Something had stilled itself within me and around me.

After that night, I never really saw John again. Every once in a while, one of the lost children might appear. The spirits I met in the mountains don't come around anymore. The plant elementals come when I call to them, and my shaman—well, he is always there when I need him. Alexis hangs around me often. She actually was around me as I wrote this book and was present when her sister Ceara was diagnosed with heart failure. My shaman and all those in heaven knew beforehand that Ceara would take ill. They also knew that I would be calling on the plant spirits.

A lot of miracles happened when Alexis crossed over. She was given life, a life beyond the veil without suffering. The miasm no longer holds any power over me, and I was initiated into the spiritual world of plants and plant gods. I was accepted as one of their own, still low on the totem pole, but granted privileges within their world. My body had shifted. I have very little reaction each year when they spray the pesticides. Changes also took place within my immediate family. Looking back, it all sometimes seems like a dream, but when I hear those footsteps behind me in the ethers, I know that my shaman still walks behind me. I'm blessed to share in a world where miracles really do happen, and where the natural world is a big part of that!

PART 2

*Enter into the
Divine Nature of Plants*

10
The Divine Nature of Plants

The essence of humankind and our birthright stems from God like the leaves of the many flowers, plants, and trees of creation. In the manifestation of a living thing, the miracle of grace showers spiritual energy onto the earth plane to harvest fruit of the Divine womb. This has come to be called a plant. The seedlings and flowers it bears represent the many aspirations toward the Divine. In our search for meaning, the relationship to God has been marked by our relationship to the Earth and all of its creatures. One may find it easier to communicate with the living things of God than directly with the Creator. In connecting with the many plants and flowers, one finds the mystical aspect of the Divine grounded in a way that resembles the physicality of our survival on Earth. Thus, we mirror the plant in its earth form as self and in the Divine form as God and Goddess. The earth form takes on all of the characteristics that we do.

The plant begins as a seed, as does an embryo in the womb. Through nourishment, the seed grows and matures and is able to walk its own path. It needs sunlight, food, appropriate shelter or settings, and love. It is nourished by respect, appreciation, and acknowledgment. Within the essence of the plant are the mysteries of God. Its innate spiritual and medicinal healing abilities are forthright and honored as part of its core. The spiritual connection to the Divine, to the God within, is so apparent that the soul line of the plant stems from deep within the earth and reaches far into the heavens. We, as humans, get nourished from the moment we are in our mother's wombs; our spirits get nourished even before then. With the right tender loving encouragement, we are given the tools to walk this path in life. Our soul line also stems from deep within the earth and reaches far into the heavens. Only we have hidden ourselves behind veils of tears and shadows, afraid to shine in the image and likeness of the Divine that is inherent within each one of us. The plants have much to teach us.

> Little flower—
> but if I could understand
> what you are, root and all, and all in all.
> I should know what God is and man is.
> *Alfred, Lord Tennyson 1809–92*

In holding the space for evolutionary growth, the plants show us the road that leads to the kingdom of God. Their stems represent our grounding, our connection to Mother Earth, the placenta that nourished us from inside the womb and still energetically and spiritually nurtures us through life. It is that part of the plant that sustains it, that part that feeds us physically and holds the space for us to find our way back to Spirit, within, above, and beyond. The sepals of the plant protect the gentle bud until it opens and expands itself to receive the complete blessings of the Divine. In choosing to live as human beings and learning to love, the outer shell we carry serves as our protection. In remembrance that all things turn to dust and eventually return to earth, the spirit always returns home. Following the way of grace is the route the spirits of plants and humans take. Grace is that miracle of life where the energies of God meet the energies of humanity. Within that realm begins the circle of life and the journey back to our essence. We call on grace to nourish our souls and help us to make clear the road ahead. In working with the plants, their connection to God is never underestimated. The sacred power is utilized to bring joy, beauty, and healing into the world.

Like us, the plants have many aspirations, which are represented by the many petals and leaves. Their petals represent the many layers of the human energy field and the various levels of evolution and enlightenment. There are many paths that lead to Spirit, and each path has a different story to tell, a different lesson to learn. On each path, there are physical, emotional, and spiritual relationships that are created to serve our highest purpose. Each of the petals resonates with a part of a life story and with a vibrational frequency of light needed for healing. The plant's work on the earth plane is to make the connection between the earth story and the light just as it is our work to do so. The sepals we carry are reminders and guides that carry us through this life to bring us back to the light, which *never* left us.

Each plant is imbued with both feminine and masculine aspects of the Divine, each aspect learning to be in relationship with the other. It is the honoring and integration of each aspect that brings unity to the plant life-force. This unity gives the plant strength to move and grow in the direction of God and a purpose for fulfilling its mission. The life-force of the whole plant has the capabilities of delivering the graces of Spirit to itself, the Earth, and to many of us. The interrelationship of the plant kingdom represents the relationship we have with the many different cultures here on Earth, the many faces of God. That is the beauty of life. All of the living creatures that come from love are unique in their own forms. In being unique, we are all one and connected with tiny strands of light, each of which breathes fire and air into the collective consciousness. We all work together to heal humanity and each kingdom, be it animal, mineral, or plant; we all serve Spirit in the same capacity. Truth follows energy.

Energy follows love. Love follows oneness. In maintaining the truth that we are all one, we become part of the plant world and receive as many teachings as our consciousness will allow. My intention in this work is to bring you some of them.

> The kiss of the sun for pardon
> The song of the birds for mirth
> One is nearer God's heart in the Garden
> Than anywhere else on Earth.
> *Dorothy Francis Gurney*

The evolution of plants is not a mystery. It is we ourselves who continue to create the illusion. The plants exist to teach us. They are like enlightened beings who choose to forgo Nirvana in order to remain here to teach us the Way, only their way is one of humility, simplicity and eternal truth. Most plants have markings on their leaves, petals, or stems that show us the many times we humans have forgotten the truth. In a way, they bear the scars and joys of human evolution. They still choose to thrive and give love when we ask for it. In their serving of Spirit, they remain humble to their teachings and continue to offer us new ways to heal.

These ways open us to a new world of healing. The Spirit, leaves, roots, flowers, and other parts of the plant are used to make medicines to heal us at the different levels of our being. They heal vibrationally, as our spirits work in mirrored relationships to those of the plant kingdom. When we need assistance on the physical, emotional, mental, or spiritual levels, the plant can access different healing states of consciousness in order to produce the right remedies for us. These remedies work in conjunction with the desired healing intent while simultaneously effecting healing in other parts of ourselves. For example, if one has lung congestion, the plant will harvest a remedy not only for the lungs, but also for the connecting emotional and spiritual issues that are in relationship with the physical malady. The beauty of this method is that most of the plants willingly share this information. All one has to do is ask the spirit of the plant.

> The Divine nature is simple, pure, unique, immutable, unalterable, ever abiding in the same way, and never goes outside of itself. It is utterly immune to any participation in evil and thus possesses the good without limit, because it can see no boundary to its own perfection.
>
> *Gregory of Nyssa*

The Plant Spirit

Each plant is like nectar of the Divine and has a spirit as we do. Its soul is three-dimensional, and the realm of the spirit unfolds as such. The lower self of the plant spirit is the plant itself in physical form. Its higher self is the God-self. The middle way is the realm of the plant spirits and devas, the many beings who help to activate the miraculous healing abilities of the plant kingdom. When working with the plant, we are working with its spirit. Just as we need our spirits to breathe life, so does the plant world to also sustain itself.

The spirits and devas are very interesting in that they maintain some sort of personality within their working dimensions. The plant spirits may appear as animals, beings, symbols, and many other things. These are the beings we call on and rely upon for assistance. Each spirit resonates at the same frequency as the plant and also serves as its protector. These spirits are messengers between the two worlds, different dimensions, and alternate realties. They bring our prayers from the earth level to the Divine to be heard and answered. In forming a relationship with plants, we form a relationship with the spirit world. The plant kingdom is a very safe way to open doors into that world. When we heal at the human level, we always work with Spirit. In working with the plants, it is the same. In having our prayers answered, the aspect of grace at the earth level works divinely in our lives.

Each spirit has something to share with us about the world and how we have evolved as a healing species. In exploring plant spirits, we acknowledge their gifts to our growth as a whole, and we work in communion with them to continue to heal ourselves. As we heal ourselves, we heal each other. What reflects within, reflects without. In healing each other, we heal the Earth and all the manifestations of God. This of course makes all the plant spirits very happy. We learn to respect Mother Nature, and the law of reciprocity comes into being. "Do unto others as you would like to have them do unto you." This rings true for the plant kingdom as well as for God's other creations.

We create beliefs and untruths about who we are and how we are supposed to live. When one begins working with plant spirits, our untruths become clearer, as does the Way. In all of our relationships on the Earth, we strive to know ourselves and Spirit. The next time you look at a plant, try to tune in to the spirit that watches over it and nourishes it.

> Keep watch over them and do not lose them; you will be connected to Absolute unity above, and the vitality of absolute unity is connected to heaven.
>
> *Huainanzi*

Plant Spirit Healing

A few years ago in the late evening, I was walking with a friend in her garden. I glanced over at a certain plant that caught my attention. The energy around it was radiant, and the light permeated the other plants surrounding it. I walked over to it and asked my friend what it was. "Lamb's ear," she said, and I knew by the vibration and light that it had something special to share. I didn't know anything about it, but by just tuning in to it, a story began to unfold. I started receiving impressions on its spiritual healing qualities, and I knew I needed to tincture the healing properties into an essence. She graciously showed me how. Upon giving thanks to the plant for sharing its medicine, three fireflies came fluttering around me in acknowledgment of the exchange.

In healing with plants, we are working with two aspects, the vibration and the spirit of the plant. When we call upon the spirit, we immediately come into Divine relationship with the plant kingdom, and the powers of that spirit manifest in the healing properties of the plant. The spirit gives to the plant its healing qualities and will also share with you the ways and times of optimal harvesting and healing. Each spirit has a vibration that filters through the physical plant body and emanates outward. The plant graciously accepts its path and work ahead and embodies the healing energies of that spirit. Its vibration also resonates with the emotional, physical, and spiritual aspects of the person it will assist in the healing process. When one needs healing from a plant, if one just listens, the right plant will show itself.

Plant spirit healing works with light energy and is a vibrational healing process. Each living thing is made up of light of many frequencies or vibrations. Denser vibrations become manifest into form and matter. The light around living things has different layers within which are qualities that resonate with the various dimensions of our spirits. One layer will resonate with the physical body, another will resonate with the emotional body, and so on. The layers are all interconnected, and one layer cannot be affected without affecting the others, as one bodily dimension cannot be healed without healing the others. In working with one layer, the vibrational healing will emanate to the other ones. When we work with plants, or the medicines that source from them, we open ourselves to receive the vibrational healing that directs itself to the place we need it most.

As Buddha said, "To walk safely through the maze of human life, one needs the light of wisdom and the guidance of virtue."

I recall working with a client a while back and calling upon the medicine of the plant spirits for assistance. She was a young woman in her midforties who came to see me about a serious case of internal inflammation and scarring. The pain became so intense that it disrupted her lifestyle on many levels. In beginning our work, I shared with her the different reasons for her illness that were communicated to me. We reflected on the emotional and spiritual aspects of the challenge she was working with and explored ways to heal and bring grace to this. In working with her digestive system, I saw in her energy field and empathically felt an intense pain in a different area of her body. I mentioned it to her. The woman recalled a time in her life when she was injured in that area. The energy around the injury remained with her for years and carried itself in her energy field, in her emotional and mental bodies, and in her spiritual body. On the physical level, the energy of the injury traveled down the nerve pathways into the stomach, causing it to be weakened. I was given the remedies that she was to use. One of them was a tonifier of a bark that worked with different organ systems, and the other was a tea that was to be made from boiling certain herbs. A few of the herb names came through, and some of them were shown to me in their natural state. It took me a few days to obtain some of the herbs, and I still wasn't familiar with some whose "pictures" were shown to me. I asked my teachers on the inner planes and the plant spirits to help bring in the vibration of the plants that were needed. In response, the healing energies of the medicines were immediately sent along with the spirits.

Upon her next visit, the pain had dissipated. I know that whatever healing needed to happen was because of the Divine connection.

Working with the physical plant itself is not at all necessary to work with its spirit medicine. Since we are working with Spirit and its vibration, many times we can just call on Spirit to hear our prayers. I suggest taking medicines internally only when the energy of the illness has permeated the tissues and cells of the human body. One can meditate or journey with a plant and obtain its healing graces as though its medicine were taken internally.

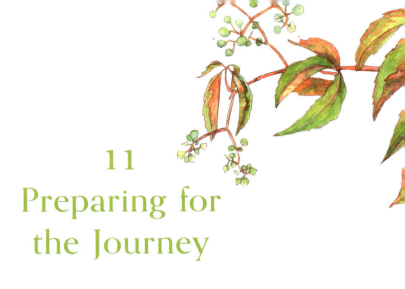

11
Preparing for the Journey

Upon starting your journey, make sure you are in a comfortable space. Be it a place in nature or your own living room, have all the tools you need to feel safe and ready for your meditation. Tools might include music, a cushion to sit on, a drum or rattle, a notebook for recording your thoughts, some prayers, an offering of gratitude, and the plant spirit with whom you want to get acquainted. Sound is very useful in that it brings one more easily to altered states of consciousness.

Begin with an invocation prayer. Offer the journey in the light of the highest good and thank Spirit for its willingness to participate. Always call on your teachers for assistance and protection, be it any tradition, any path. When you travel into the spirit world, there are certain things you need to be aware of and protection is necessary, which may come from prayer, burning an herb or resin such as sage or copal, or from a ritual, or blessing. When I do this work, I call on my guiding teachers in the spirit world. In exploring your spiritual work and inner process, always call on beings with whom you resonate and feel safe. Because I am working with a living creation of the Earth, it is customary to honor that element, its traditions, and spiritual energies. Calling in the four elements of air, fire, water, and earth respects our connection to the Mother.

After your guides and teachers are present, you may ask the plant spirit with whom you would like to work to become present. It is not necessary for you to have the plant with you in physical form, although working next to it is very magical and powerful. A vision of the plant will do as well. It might take a while for the plant spirit to make itself known. Like all spirits of the light, they want to make sure your intention is clear. Tell the spirit you request its presence for healing purposes and are honored by its willingness to be with you. Once you feel a presence, you may begin your work. If you have the plant within your reach, ask to touch a part of it and begin to feel its physical characteristics. If you are holding a vision, look closely at the different parts of the plant. See if you can "feel" it with your vision. Notice the texture and the shape of the leaves. Look for flowers. Hold the stem gently. Get a feel for the physicality of the plant structure and see how it mirrors the human body. The closer you get to becoming one with the plant, the sooner the plant spirit will identify itself. If you are familiar with journeying and working in the spirit world, the spirit might come to you more readily. As you embody the physicality and energetics of the plant matrix, become aware of the sensations in your body. Notice what parts of you—organs, bones, tissues, and muscles—are experiencing different sensations as you work with them. By being in physical energetic resonance, your body begins to mirror the maladies that the plant spirit heals. Journey deeper. Ask the plant what parts of its physicality will help to heal those sensations you are experiencing. You might be surprised at what you hear. You will receive information on how to bring the spirit of the plant into your body. This is a good time to record some of your thoughts. Thank the plant for teaching you about how it physically heals, and ask it to now help you tune in to the emotional body.

> **Do not treat lightly the things that enter a person's life ... receive them for what they are and then try to make them fit tools for enlightenment.**
>
> **Lord Buddha**

Clear your body of the physical sensations and tune in to your emotional being. Begin by gently breathing into your lower abdomen. Breathe in through your nose and exhale through your mouth. Do this a number of times to bring your consciousness into another state of awareness. Let your emotions be safely present within you so as to bring awareness to that part of you we are working with. Greet them and let them move through you so you become a clear channel to allow the plant spirit to share with you its emotional healing qualities. When you are ready, ask the plant spirit to share with you how the plant heals the emotional body. Tune in to yourself as you do this. You will begin to notice emotions surfacing in your body. They may be the same ones as before or different ones. They may be new. Are you experiencing grief, joy, anger, forgiveness? What healing qualities does this plant and spirit offer you? Remember that each plant will offer something different to everyone. One plant may heal grief in one person, while healing anger in another. Each spirit adapts itself to the environment and the person with whom it is communicating.

When you feel complete with the emotional healing experience, thank the plant spirit once again for its guidance. As before, clear your body by breathing into your lower abdomen, breathing in through your nose and exhaling through your mouth, and honoring and detaching from all that is moving through you at the moment so that you become a clear channel.

When you are ready, tune in to your spirit. Envision yourself as a ball of light, endlessly flowing out into the universe, connected with all things, radiating loving kindness to the Earth and all of her creatures. Feel your soul line stemming from deep within the earth and reaching far into the heavens. Know that you are one with the Divine. When you have come to that place, ask the plant and spirit to share with you their spiritual healing qualities. How can they help you heal your life on the spiritual level? How can they help you find or rekindle your connection to God? Listen to what the spirit tells you. You will begin to notice higher vibrations of spiritual energy working through and around you. You will begin to feel healing on a different level. Take as much time as you need with yourself in this place. The spirit and plant are healing your spirit, which in turn, will heal your physical and emotional bodies.

> From Wakan Tanka, the Great Mystery, comes all power. It is from Wakan Tanka that the holy man has wisdom and the power to heal and make holy charms. Man knows that all healing plants are given by Wakan Tanka, therefore they are holy.
> *Flat Iron, Oglala Sioux Chief*

When you are complete with this part, acknowledge the spirit and plant for their assistance. If you haven't already seen the plant spirit clearly, ask for it to make itself known to you, if that is to be seen in alignment with the highest will. If the spirit feels it would serve you, you will make its visual acquaintance. Be patient. As on the human level, some spirits need to create a resonance of trust before showing themselves.

You have now finished journeying, and it is time to come to a completion and a letting go. I like to offer a prayer of thanks. Saying a simple thank-you from the heart or a prayer of gratitude in the tradition that you resonate with works wonderfully. Thank the spirit of the plant and the plant itself for joining you. Also thank your guides and teachers for protecting and guiding this journey. Part of giving thanks is to make an offering. An offering is something from the heart, be it a prayer, thanks, or praise to the spirit keepers and creations of the earth. You might use something from your person, like a strand of hair, or bury something sentimental that belongs to you. You might want to burn incense or resin again. The earth also likes sweet-tasting things.

After your offering, bring your awareness back to your being, and I encourage you to write down some notes of your journey. I hope you enjoy your adventure!

12
The Healing Dimensions and Prayer

I worked with a woman who came to see me while she was very sick. She was thirty years of age, with a history of environmental illness and energy sensitivity. She had an infection that had run a course through the urinary tract, the intestines, and the rectum and had left her with a fever for over two months. She had difficulty breathing and walking. The doctors couldn't find very much, and she explored many different pathways to healing. As we began our work together, the sacred space that was created was filled with shamans and medicine people from the outer planes. They came to share with me some of the reasons for her illness. We were transported to another lifetime where the shamans showed me that this woman suffered from a severe case of tuberculosis and parasitic infection. Her legs had boils on them and were bleeding from the infection. She was ridden with fever and dementia. She was being helped by Indigenous healers and friends around her. From the looks of things, she wasn't faring so well. The energy pattern set up in that former incarnation stayed with her through this lifetime and embedded itself in her energy field. Through different experiences in this lifetime, the old energy matrix became stronger and intruded into her physical body. Some of her karmic issues from this pattern became obvious, as did the emotional healing from that former life that needed to take place.

In order to help heal the energy around her current physical illness, we had to work energetically and spiritually to heal the karma from the past life. After the shamans showed me her experience, they worked with the plant spirits to heal the woman in her past incarnation. They began with special prayers to invoke the help of the spirits of the medicines they were to use with the woman. They took leaves of some plant and crushed them into tiny pieces in a bowl. They boiled the leaves in water to make a tea. They also spread some of the leaves over the boils of the woman. They continually prayed to the plant spirits for the medicine to work. When the tea was ready, they drank it first and spit it over the woman's body three times, drenching her from head to toe. They seemed to use this method when serious illness was present. Then they gently raised her head so she could sip some tea from the bowl to help cast out any demons internally. They waved their hands over the woman's body in a fanlike procedure, as though waving the energy of the illness off the body and continued with their prayers to the plant spirits. Cloths were laid on the woman's head and body to bring down her fever and cool her from the heat of the infection, drawing out many toxins. The shamans took about fifteen minutes to do this healing procedure. The woman began to experience different sensations in her body in this reality while the shamans were working in the other. I began to notice the energies clearing off her bodies in both that incarnation and the present. When the work was complete, both beings were more peaceful. The shamans closed their healing with prayers of gratitude, as I offered my own to those who had come to help. The woman noticed a big shift in her present body and felt a weight lift off her that she had carried for a long time. Her body and spirit then began to heal on a different level.

I shared this story to show you the powerful effects of using the plant spirits and their medicines for healing illness that originates at the spiritual level. Sometimes the origin may be in another incarnation, yet still affect the present-day reality.

The plant spirits can effect change within the spiritual, emotional, and physical states of being. All of our unhealed thoughts, emotions, experiences, incarnations, and karma are carried in our energy fields until the vibration is cleared with our continued personal evolution. We clear those stagnant energies by transmuting them to the higher vibrational source from which they came. When patterns stay in the energy field for lifetimes, they can cause a number of imbalances within us. Purification happens when the energies become transmuted and we grow closer in alignment to Source.

A few years ago, I assisted on a case where a young woman was going through a lot of emotional upheaval. The practitioner working with this woman was having some challenges with this person's personality. I asked permission to see if I could "tune in" and see what was happening in this person's energy consciousness. I was able to see that she had suffered much sexual trauma and neglect during her childhood. As an adult, she was stuck in a pattern of identifying with abuse and abandonment and testing others to make sure they wouldn't leave her. Also in her field were many entities that were feeding upon her self-inflicted patterns of emotional abuse. What was transpiring between client and practitioner was that the entities were attacking both the practitioner and the client during the work, so it was difficult for the client to put the entities into perspective and let them go. This situation was also testing the practitioner's own boundaries about needing the client to take responsibility for herself at whatever level she could. Every time the practitioner found himself trying to affirm his boundaries and work with his client, the entities only seemed to get stronger, furthered by the client's own need to emotionally put herself down. I suggested to the practitioner, as it came to me, to call upon the spirit of black cohosh, and I explained to him how the plant spirit energetically aligned with the physical, emotional, and spiritual challenges that faced his client and how it might not only help the entities to find the light, but it might also bring some peace of mind to his client. Sometime later, the practitioner called to thank me, letting me know that when he called upon the black cohosh spirit, the entities left his client's energy field and a great healing session resulted. Black cohosh is excellent in assisting with trauma of this kind, and I would recommend it for similar cases, both in calling upon the spirit and in using an essence of the plant homeopathically.

Each plant in this book has a section that was communicated on its spiritual and emotional healing properties. Each spirit has vibrational qualities that resonate with the vibrations of different emotions. When you call in the spirit to work with an emotion, its healing vibration will match that of the emotion and the positive and negative poles will neutralize each other. In simple terms, light will dissipate the darkness and peace will find its way within. The spirit will only work to strengthen what you already have.

When spiritual issues arise in the energy body, the plant spirit accesses the energies of its higher self to resonate with those that need healing. Spiritual issues may include karmic patterns, negative spirits in the energy field, "curses," and so on. Those issues are addressed at the heart-and-soul level of a person, and the plant surrenders much of its physical body in working under these circumstances. The light from the spirit filters into the soul line of the person and permeates from the center outward, affecting the various layers of the energy field. It creates a solid formation similar to a healing grid and holds the template in place until all that needs to happen for the person does so. This is all in accordance with the will of the highest good.

In the physical healing state, imbalances in the body manifest first in the energy field. Through challenges, lifetime experiences, and holding patterns in the etheric body, illness arises as a means to signal the unconscious to awaken. When a plant spirit works vibrationally to heal the physical body, it becomes denser in energy and strengthens its own field to be able to work at this level. Its own cells and tissues become imbued with nutrients that manifest from Spirit. The energies of these nutrients surround the energy field of the plant and create an energetic transfusion into the person receiving the healing medicine.

> We bow mind and heart in prayer before God.
> We silence the outer self and banish worldly matters
> and thoughts. With deep and compassionate love
> for all mankind we await the incoming of the spirit.
> Spiritual power now encompasses us. Steadily, quietly,
> deeply, we breathe in the Spirit of God . . . we pray.
> Fill you, oh Spirit, fill us, fill us, and bless our
> endeavor to heal.
>
> *White Eagle*

Healing and Prayer

When we heal with plant spirits, commitment to our evolution is of utmost importance. The healings work as much as we allow them to and insofar as we have faith. Faith is the necessary ingredient for all graces to ground themselves in physical reality. We need a willingness to explore our realities, to look deeply within ourselves and find the original sources of our wounding. The journey requires gentleness, compassion toward oneself, nonjudgment, and the ability to let go. When we surrender to the process, a miraculous partnership begins to unfold between yourself and the world of plant spirits.

In this new partnership, the plant and its spirit form energetic bonds of light with you. Your energies become merged, and the plant spirit helps the plant adapt to your vibration and assists you in receiving it. The partnership is a very nurturing one, as the plant senses your healing needs on all levels. Sometimes the plant takes on the person's illness as it is better able than we are to hand it over to the spirit world or to Mother Earth. In giving permission to the plant spirits to carry out their work, we create the space for Divine Union and mutual reciprocity.

It is essential to let go of how we think they will assist us in our healing and what the outcome will be. We might need assistance with a form of cancer and the plant spirit may instruct the healing energies of the plant to heal anger issues that stem from childhood. Trusting in Divine Providence creates a healthy healing relationship between you and the plant, and letting go of your wounding with great compassion assists the process even further.

The following is an anonymous prayer that I use to remind myself of the journey we take with the plant spirits and the medicine we receive.

> *When the wind blows, that is my medicine.*
> *When it rains, that is my medicine.*
> *When it hails, that is my medicine.*
> *When it becomes clear after a storm,*
> *That is my medicine.*

The Power of Prayer in Healing

Life is a prayer. Every aspect of creation is, in essence, a prayer when we enter into conscious relationship with it. In working with nature, we enter into prayer the moment we acknowledge the divine attributes and healing qualities of the plant. Our relationship to the plant becomes the vehicle for our evolution as spiritual beings.

The action of grounding the prayer manifests in the healing work we do with the plants. Intention is vital, as it sets up the space for the energy to unfold and work in accordance with Divine Providence. An energetic matrix through which the spiritual energies come is formed by the ways in which we observe, see, touch, taste, and smell the living things around us. Respect for the plant and its spirit is very important, for they are the doorkeepers that lead to the higher dimensions. They are the ones who bring our prayers to the Highest Will.

In praying with the plant, we are saying, "I need your assistance. I am ready to receive whatever is necessary for my healing and growth. I surrender my intentions in the light of the highest good and will do my part in helping myself heal."

When we offer prayers, we are saying that we have faith in the miraculous healing abilities of the plant and its spirit. We are saying that *we believe*! In offering prayer at the beginning of our work, we align ourselves with the higher vibrational healing energies that come from Spirit. We invite Spirit to come into our lives and heal us. The exchange between us and the plant world is sacred and unique to each individual. We are not welcoming a new friend into our lives; we are welcoming ourselves back home.

Gratitude is the greatest prayer we can offer to Spirit and to the earth. Always remember we are never alone, and we have many assistants and guides in every aspect of our lives. It is humbling to wake up and be grateful for having life and the beauty of creation that surrounds us. In expressing gratitude, we are acknowledging the greater workings in our lives that carry us along the way. Having gratitude also fosters a sense of compassion and humility for life's mysteries, the world and all of its peoples.

In working with the plants in this book, a prayer was communicated to each plant spirit to access higher states of consciousness to effect healing. The prayer reflected the vibration of the spirit and the energies of spiritual, emotional, and physical healing. These powerful prayers are doorways to the Divine and hold the space for the light to come through.

A sample of a Mayan prayer follows . . .

In the name of the Father, the Son, and the Holy Spirit (or insert name of your deity). I give thanks to the spirit of this plant, and I have faith with all my heart that you will help me to heal the sickness of (insert your name or name of the patients or the people). Amen.

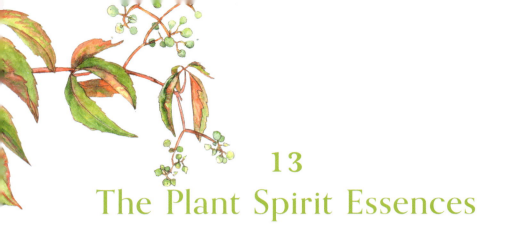

13
The Plant Spirit Essences

At the onset of this book, while I was working with plants and their spirits, it became clear that remedies for healing various ailments energetically were to be communicated. Different plant parts were to be used in various ways, and plant essences from nature were to be made. The remedies in this book are not cures. They work energetically to heal issues in the emotional, physical, and spiritual states of being. With each plant spirit, there is a section titled "The Physical Healing Properties," within which are listed physical ailments and how to use essences and various plant parts to heal energetically. The essences contain the vibrational healing energy of each plant spirit.

With these new teachings, the intent is to assist you in creating a healing relationship between yourself and the earth and in making your own medicines from nature. When you put into your body a substance of your own creation and energy, you nurture yourself with your own divine essence.

How to Make Your Own Plant Spirit Essence

In making an essence for your personal use, the most important tools are prayers, love, and gratitude and your relationship with the plant spirit upon journeying. If you choose to make an essence to take internally, trust the plant spirit to tell you the most fertile time for harvesting the necessary plant part to help you with your creation. I have listed the plant parts that are to be used with the plants mentioned in this book.

You will need spring water; alcohol, such as vodka or brandy, as a preserving agent; the part of the plant used for the medicine; a clear glass bowl; and your intuition. You will be guided as to the part of the day in which you are called to harness the healing energies of the plant spirit. I suggest that you create a sacred space and begin your journey with the plant spirit there. You might want to make your creation in the sun, in the night with the energy of the moon, or in a special meditation room. Take the part of the plant you will be using and immerse it in a small, clear bowl filled with spring water. Intuit the amount of time needed for the healing energy of the plant and spirit to imbue the water. When the energies of both have aligned with the water and have been blessed by the Divine, your water is now potentized and becomes a plant spirit essence. Place your essence in a secure, clean, one-ounce bottle in a proportion of four parts essence to one part alcohol, and your process is complete. The alcohol secures the earth element, while the plant spirit essence holds the space for the etheric. In making the essences, much love, prayer, and vibrational plant spirit energy helps to create these medicines of the earth and sky.

Plant spirit essences have no adverse side effects. However, like all plant medicines, they allow for the natural healing process of the self to unfold. This may cause suppressed physical symptoms to appear, or symptoms might become exacerbated as in a healing crisis before shifting in the body. Unfamiliar and unexpressed emotions and all forms of toxicity may also surface as the body and its various levels become healed.

There are many instances where I suggest using an herbal massage oil. There are two ways to accomplish this.

1. Macerate (mash) about 2 oz. of dried herb, or twice that amount of fresh herb with a mortar and pestle. Place the herb in a one-pint lidded jar and fill with the recommended oil. Let the mixture stand in a warm place for three days. Strain and bottle the oil, and it is ready to use.
2. Combine the herbs and oil in a pot that is large enough to hold both. Heat the mixture gently for one hour, keeping it uncovered. The temperature should remain under 200° F. Strain and bottle the mixture when cooled.

To make an infusion or tea, bring one pint of water to a full boil in a medium-size pot, then remove it from the burner. Put about two cups of the dried herb (more if fresh) in the boiled water and cover the pot tightly. Allow it to steep for ten to fifteen minutes depending on how strong you want it.

The following plant parts were used to make the essences and remedies in this book. I ask you to follow your own intuition and guidance from the plant spirits. Use whichever plant parts you are drawn to using. Consciousness changes every moment, as do the physical, emotional, and spiritual realms of our being and the collective universe. The vibrations of the plants and their parts will mirror that.

Angelica–leaf
Astragalus–leaf
Black Cohosh–leaf
Blessed Thistle–leaf
Calendula–leaf
Chamomile–leaf and flower
Clematis–leaf
Dandelion–leaf and flower
Feverfew–leaf
Lamb's Ear–leaf

Lavender–leaf
Lemon Balm–leaf
Licorice–leaf
Lilac–leaf and flower
Marshmallow–leaf
Motherwort–leaf
Mugwort–leaf
Mullein–leaf
Nettles–leaf
Poke–plant spirit only

Pulsatilla–leaf, flower, and stem
Red Clover–leaf
Rosemary–leaf
Rue–leaf
Sage–leaf

Skullcap–leaf
St. John's Wort–leaf
Violet–leaf
Wormwood–leaf
Yarrow–leaf

PART 3

The Plants, the Spirits, and Their Healing

14
Introducing the Plants

I have communicated with the spirit world since I was a child, but it was much later that I began to consciously communicate with the plant realm. One of the spirits that has guided me in my healing work and life has been a Japanese healer, herbalist, teacher, and friend from the sixteenth century. His knowledge of plant medicine is vast, and his techniques for healing with them are many. I have given him the name "Honored One," and he was the impetus for my writing this section of the book. Part of his practice was to communicate plants and herbs to me with directions for preparation and usage. He works very sacredly with plant medicine and energy consciousness, and I have learned much from him about healing and the use of this plant medicine. Sometimes he would want me to work with the plant in its natural state. He would communicate this by just showing me the leaf, flower, or whole plant itself. It became challenging when my lack of plant identification and formal training would leave me searching for the plant he meant. I wanted to learn more and understand the way he did. And thus, a way was shown, a way in which we can all learn to communicate with the plant realm.

I was guided to write this part of the book on the spiritual, emotional, and physical healing properties of plants. Spirits communicated the information through various intuitive means. What manifested out of my apprenticeship with this work are novel and ancient teachings on working with plant medicines. In this section are thirty plants whose words needed to be heard. I was given the plants to work with.

I journeyed with the plants, and their spirits came to me and shared their stories. I sat in meditation with each plant as its spirit told me of its emotional, spiritual, and healing properties. Some of this information was communicated through clairaudience, and as the vibration of the physical illness passed through my body, other information passed to me kinesthetically. Instructions followed on how to make a plant spirit essence with certain plant parts. With each plant came a prayer—an invocation and gesture of gratitude for the work and knowledge that was shared.

> *Earth ourselves,*
> *breathe and awaken,*
> *leaves are stirring,*
> *all things moving,*
> *new day coming,*
> *life renewing.*
>
> PAWNEE PRAYER

I was told the best time for communicating with each plant spirit. Some days I would wake up and just know that it was time to partake in their healing medicine. The vibration and peak healing frequency varied from plant to plant. When I communicated with a certain plant spirit, I would work near the plant and ask its permission to harvest and hold the parts that were to be used for healing purposes. At the end of the communication, I noticed that the parts that I held were withered and that the life-force of the plant had passed through my body, showing me its energies and the illness it healed. Their nectar became aligned with my life-force, as it is with all living things. After giving its life and healing, the plant spirit would leave and that plant part would literally die. I was moved by this in appreciation, and I wondered how we could honor the earth and harvest the medicines sparingly so as to avoid unnecessary plant-life destruction. Upon completing my work with each plant, I again offered my gratitude and devotion.

Despite the physical death of the plant parts, the plant spirit remains alive and vibrant! It is this spirit that nurtures new growth to come. Each plant part has served its purpose as part of Divine Providence and the plant will regenerate with the help of its spirit. After experiencing the unconditionally loving generosity of each plant that I worked with, I placed the withered part next to the plant from which it came, so Mother Earth could cradle it gently in her arms.

With the Earth in such a state of change and unrest, and with many species of plants being overharvested and dying out, we need to search for new ways of utilizing with care and gentleness our most precious resources and earth's creations. The evolution of time and consciousness is rapidly changing. The Earth itself, its people, and their illnesses are also changing in matter, vibration, and essence. The way we use medicines has to change if we are ever to heal ourselves and the Earth and preserve our resources. If we can begin to use medicines vibrationally, it will do much to preserve our resources and effect healing in a more precise way. When you work vibrationally with plant medicine, you use the plants in conjunction with the vibration of what you are trying to heal, whatever its level. In this way, you utilize less of the plant and more of its spirit. You will also begin to utilize plant medicines differently. Preparation methods and best times to use the medicine will be communicated to you by the plant spirits. Remember, less is more. I have often seen that a few drops of an earth medicine taken in accordance with a body's needs can have more of an effect than plant-derived medicine taken at full dosage.

In working with the earth in this new but ancient way, you will learn to truly respect the plants, their medicine, and their healing powers. You will also give yourself and the land time to produce healthier gardens, and you will create medicines that will benefit all of humankind.

> I love plants because of the way babies and old people touch them, and the look they bring to a lover's eye. I love how each smells a little different from the rest.
> — *Jesse Wolf Hardin*

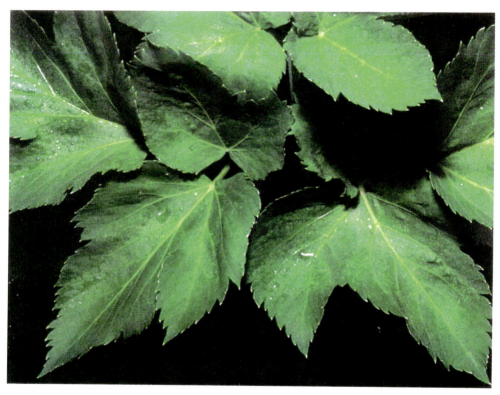

Angelica

Plant Spirit Prayer

Sages of old, bestow unto us your blessings of guidance and protection.

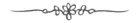

Angelica
(*Angelica archangelica*)

My Experience with This Plant Spirit

When calling on the plant spirit, not one, but many came to assist angelica. They looked like children, young girls and boys; only they are old souls and have lived in the spirit world for centuries. They possess gifts of magic and wizardry, and their role is to protect all men, women, and children from harm. Since they cannot leave their dimension, they harvest many angelica plants on Earth to do their work for them. Through ritual, they imbue the plants with special powers to protect and heal us.

The Spiritual and Emotional Properties

Angelica is a protective plant. It secures one's boundaries. It protects against negative influences, spells, and curses. It assists those who cannot stand up for themselves and who are prone to vulnerability. It acts as a filter for those who communicate with the spirit world and protects the psychic field.

Angelica represents the duality of life, the light and dark sides of nature that need to coexist in a harmonious state. Call on the spirit of the plant when one is having a nervous breakdown. It helps to alleviate severe emotional stress and loss of emotional control. It naturally numbs the emotional nervous system when it is overwhelmed. It is excellent in reducing hypersensitivity in people, especially those who are energetically sensitive.

The Physical Healing Properties

Do not use when pregnant.

- 🌿 Angelica is excellent for healing the pain of headaches: upon the onset of the pain, take 3 drops of the essence in water and sip slowly.

- 🌿 It also helps to alleviate high blood pressure: place a drop of the essence under your tongue when needed or massage a mixture of drops of the essence with almond oil onto your chest.

- 🌿 It is also excellent in healing the energy around angina and heart attacks: make a compress of fresh leaves and place on the chest area for twenty-minute intervals. Do this by moistening the leaves with a little warmed water and placing them between folded layers of cotton cloth.

- 🌿 For fevers, use the same compress and place it on the forehead until the fever is reduced.

- 🌿 For colicky babies, make a massage oil of the leaves and flowers in olive oil and massage a small amount onto their backs.

- 🌿 Angelica acts as a natural stimulant and antibiotic when used homeopathically in sick children. When the need arises, place a few drops of the essence in water for them to sip slowly. **Do not use this with young children.**

- 🌿 Angelica promotes the onset of the menstrual cycle: take 2 drops of the essence in water daily until one begins to menstruate.

- 🌿 It energetically tonifies the prostate in men and strengthens the uterus in women: place plants of angelica around you or take a drop of the essence under your tongue upon retiring. Only do this when one needs tonification in those two areas.

- It helps in extreme cases of mental handicap and nervous breakdown by calming the nervous system. Place the plants around you or take a drop of the essence in water and sip slowly.

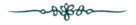

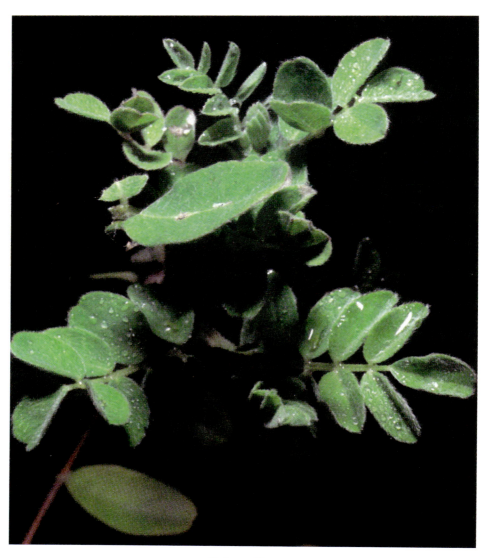

Astragalus

Plant Spirit Prayer

Gracious one. We are honored by your presence. We seek the knowledge of the mysteries of our existence. We seek to know ourselves as we are lost from our essence. Bring us home.

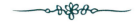

Astragalus
(Astragalus membranaceous)

My Experience with This Plant Spirit

In calling upon the spirit of the plant, an elderly Eastern man appeared to me. He is a medicine man and a magician, very mysterious in his ways and mannerisms. He doesn't say much yet has the ability to heal the broken aspects of one's soul without uttering a word. He sits in his little and very simplistic kitchen, always cooking something over the fire for those who come to visit him. And many do. They come from everywhere and are not even sure why but somehow become drawn to this mysterious man.

In envisioning him in the moment, he shows me he is with a stranger who has wandered in, looking lost and confused. The elderly man sits at his kettle stirring the mixture of hot water and herbs, one of them being the astragalus plant. Also gracefully moving in the kettle are special worms taken from his garden. These worms are gifted with medicinal and spiritual healing qualities and continue to thrive as the kettle simmers. They form a symbol around each leaf, the yin/yang symbol, and imbue the plant with masculine and feminine healing energies. When the medicine is finished cooking, the worms get replaced in the garden to rejuvenate themselves for future healings.

He offers the stranger a cup of the medicine, knowing that its power will help to bring back the man's soul that was lost so long ago. The man drinks from the cup and travels on his way, not aware of the powers that will now work in his life. The elderly medicine man sends the stranger off with a nod and returns to his simplicity. As the stranger heads down the road, if you stare closely enough, one might see a myriad of sparks floating around him as he walks and a glow in his eyes that he's been missing for a while . . . his soul has returned!

The Spiritual and Emotional Properties

Call on the spirit of the plant when one is feeling a sense of soul loss. This plant is very gifted in searching out lost souls.

Use astragalus when you are feeling emotionally shut down and cannot let anyone in . . . the plant will help you to open up. This plant spirit will always be there for you, to follow you into those deep and dark places of your life.

When your spirit leaves your body, astragalus will find it and bring it back to where it belongs. Call on the spirit of the plant when you are on a journey of discovering or rediscovering yourself.

Astragalus is excellent for helping with boundaries. It is also excellent for fostering respect for oneself and others.

The vibration of the plant is at the doorway of the lower worlds—of the physical reality—thus helping to watch over it. It is also comforting to spirits. It is very useful in long-distance healing work when working at the level of the soul.

The Physical Healing Properties

Do not use when pregnant.

- Astragalus helps to heal the energy surrounding convulsions and head injuries: make a compress of dried leaves and place over injury for thirty-minute intervals. Do this by moistening the leaves with a little warmed water and placing them between folded layers of cotton cloth.

- It also helps to balance the electrolytes in the body, as well as nourish the body when it is vitamin deficient: take 1–2 drops of the essence in water.

- It nourishes the energy of the heart: take 1–3 drops of the essence in water between 1:00 and 3:00 in the afternoon.

- It is a good remedy for balancing the nervous system: take 1 drop under the tongue upon waking. Astragalus helps when one is unable to sleep due to feeling anxiety or nervous energy: take 1 drop of the essence in water before going to bed.

- It is useful in cleansing the gallbladder and alleviating the pain of gallstones: make a compress of fresh or dried herb moistened with water. Place the herb between folded layers of cotton cloth and place over gallbladder. Massage the area first with warmed castor oil and place a heating pad on top of the compress. Do this for twenty-minute intervals.

- It also tonifies the stomach chi: make a massage oil of fresh or dried herb with wheat germ oil and massage the warmed oil onto stomach area.

- It is an excellent overall tonifier and enhances the immune system: take 3 drops of the essence in water as needed.

- Using a salve with astragalus is excellent for healing cuts and bruises. It helps to heal the energy around throat operations from the past as well as the present. Make a massage oil with the herb and olive oil and massage the warmed oil onto the throat area.

- Taking a few drops of the essence under the tongue upon waking will help to balance hormones. Calling on the plant spirit as well as bathing with the leaves is a good remedy that will balance one's masculine and feminine energies.

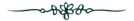

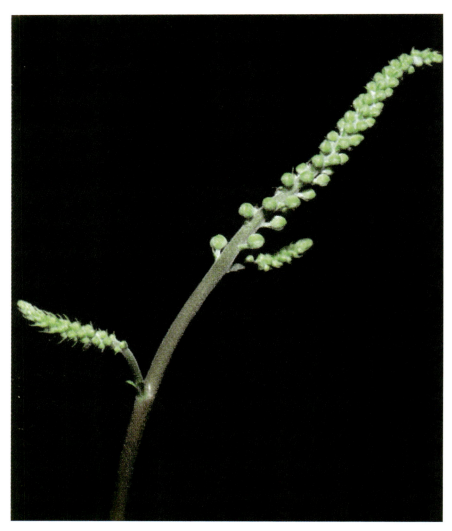

Black Cohosh

Plant Spirit Prayer

Oh sacred sounds of the earth, lull our spirits to rest upon your divine heartbeat. Take from us our pain so that you may transform it with your profound healing energy.

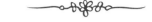

Black Cohosh
(*Cimcifuga racemosa*)

My Experience with This Plant Spirit

In calling on the plant spirit, a ceremonial dance of tribal Native American women comes into my vision. There is one among them who is a medicine woman, a healer, and a peacemaker. She leads the others in a ritual dance of prayer and offering to Mother Earth and the spirits that help her. As she chants a prayer to the earth, she motions her body upward toward the sky and then reaches downward and allows her entire being to touch and merge with the ground. In this dance, she offers herself and the soul of her womb to that of the Mother, cradling the earth as she does to find comfort and peace. As she merges herself, she takes in her hands branches of the black cohosh plant to give as an offering. Upon touching the earth, the branches become imbued with the sacred healing properties of the energies of the Mother.

The Spiritual and Emotional Properties

Call on the spirit of black cohosh to protect one from evil spirits and spirit possession. It is used in sacred ceremony to draw out spirits and ancestors from the body. It is also used as an offering to Mother Earth because of the special relationship it holds to that energy. It nourishes and honors the Mother. It is a plant that shows reverence to the wise and ancient ways of the ancestors.

Call on the spirit of the plant to assist when one has to give up a child for adoption. It will help to protect and also heal the energy surrounding it. It also is healing for the parents when a child is lost to trauma either physically, mentally, emotionally, or spiritually.

It is excellent for healing the spiritual and emotional challenges around infertility. It is called on for protection of the community. It protects against damaging fires, droughts, floods, and threat of imminent danger. It will also protect little children and animals from harm.

Call on the spirit of the plant to care for those who are entering into an uncomfortable and challenging situation. It is used to create and hold sacred space in ceremony and ritual. It is also used as an offering and gifting to the spirits for doing their work.

The Physical Healing Properties

Do not use when pregnant. It can induce miscarriage and abortion.

- Black cohosh is excellent for healing the energy around hysteria and mental illness. Call on the spirit of the plant to assist you and place many plants near you when you sleep. Adding 5–10 drops of the plant spirit essence in water a few times a day will also help.

- For uterine cramping, take 4 drops of the essence under your tongue at the onset of discomfort. Also make an oil with the leaves of black cohosh and almond oil and massage onto pelvic area.

- For nosebleeds, massage a mixture of a few drops of the essence with warmed olive oil onto your nose after the bleeding stops. It will help to heal the energy in the tissue.

- For excessive menstrual bleeding, take 3–5 drops of the essence in water upon retiring, and also massage a mixture of drops of the essence with St. John's wort oil onto the pelvic area. For extreme pain in the uterus, burn the dry leaves of black cohosh around you, and also make a poultice to place on the pelvic area. Do this by placing the fresh leaves on top of your pelvic area. Massage first with warmed olive oil. Do the same for healing the energies around fibroids, cysts, and tumors.

- To heal the energy around breast cancer, take 5 drops of the essence in water upon waking. Also place many plants around you as you sleep and massage a mixture of a few drops of the essence with almond oil onto the breast area.

- For healing the energy around cervical cancer, place a compress of the leaves of black cohosh moistened with a little warmed water on top of the pubic bone. Do this by placing the moistened leaves between layers of folded cotton cloth and leaving it on the affected area for twenty-minute intervals. Do not exceed more than twice a day.

- For bladder dysfunction in men, make an oil of the leaves and almond oil and massage the warmed oil onto the bladder area. This is best done upon retiring. It is also beneficial to place a white cloth over the bladder area while you sleep. For men who suffer from a hernia, massage drops of the essence with warmed almond oil onto the area.

- Black cohosh is excellent for heart stress and pain in the chest: make a compress of the fresh leaves moistened with water and place atop the chest area for ten-minute intervals. Do this by placing the moistened leaves between folded layers of cotton cloth. For relaxing the body, reducing stress, and calming the nervous system, place a drop of the essence under your tongue.

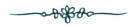

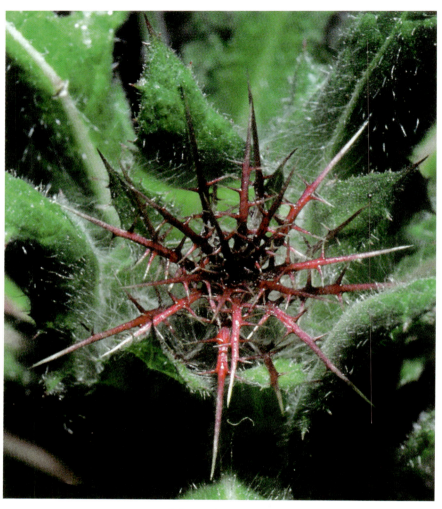

Blessed Thistle

Plant Spirit Prayer
Tender heart, take hold of those who yearn for companionship and nurturing. Bring to them a love of purity, kindness, and gentleness to be with them the rest of their days.

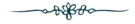

Blessed Thistle
(*Cnicus benedictus*)

My Experience with This Plant Spirit

In calling on the spirit of the plant, a wise old man appears to me. He walks with a limp and uses a cane to help him in his travels. When he is not walking, he spends much of his time in a rocker he carved out of wood. He is a quiet spirit, rocking back and forth on his chair watching the lives of many of us here. He tends to be a little grumpy at times, but don't let that fool you. Behind that grin is a spirit with a heart of gold. He is caretaker to all the humans that are left alone in this world, especially the elderly. Surrounding him are many plants of blessed thistle. They seem to have an overabundance of heart energy to give to others. Every time he sees a person whose heart is worn from feeling alone, he blesses a blessed thistle plant, and with its permission, extracts the heart energy and sends it to the person who needs healing.

The Spiritual and Emotional Properties

Call on the spirit of the plant to guide you in your prayers. It fosters self-forgiveness and brings with it compassion and absolution for all of one's past grievances and mistakes. It is useful in helping one to locate something they have lost. It soothes irritability and frustration. It assists one in concentrating on themselves and their life's work. It is used in celebrations, gatherings, and ceremony as a gifting to what is being honored. It helps to bring peace to those recovering from long-term illness.

It balances the heart energy in relationships. It is excellent in calming cranky babies and children.

Call on the spirit of the plant to help those who are codependent and tend to take on other people's issues. It will create boundaries around the heart and bring your focus back to yourself. For older people who tend to injure themselves all the time, place plants of blessed thistle around them. It will help work with the emotional energies around this. It is an energetic protector of the skeletomuscular system of the human body. Call on blessed thistle to keep company with elderly people who need attention and care.

The Physical Healing Properties

Do not use when pregnant.

- Blessed thistle is excellent for detoxifying the liver and gallbladder: make a compress of the leaves and place it over the liver and gallbladder area for twenty to thirty minutes. Do this by taking fresh or dried leaves and placing them in a generous amount of warmed castor oil. Steep the leaves for at least a half hour in the oil then place them between layers of folded cotton cloth. This is best done before retiring.

- It is a good remedy for strengthening eyesight: take a drop of the plant spirit essence under your tongue upon waking. Also place a compress of the dry leaves moistened with a touch of warmed water over the closed eyes. Do this by taking the moistened leaves and placing them between layers of folded cotton cloth. Leave on the eyes for five minutes.

- It is excellent for strengthening the immune system: place 10 drops of the essence in water once daily when you find your system weakened. It clears brain fog and improves the functioning of the brain: take 3 drops of the essence in water upon waking. It detoxifies the entire body system. Bathe with the fresh leaves of blessed thistle to provide nutrients and vitamins to the blood. Place a few drops of the essence in warmed water and drink as a tea upon waking.

- It assists in regulating the energy of the thymus gland. Massage a mixture of drops of the essence, St. John's wort oil, and almond oil onto the area of the thymus. It assists in regulating the energetics of blood pressure.

- Massage a mixture of a few drops of the essence mixed with warmed apricot oil onto the chest and heart area. It improves circulation and assists in bringing oxygen to the cells. Make an oil of the leaves of blessed thistle and almond oil and massage over the body after bathing.

- It assists in relieving menstrual cramping and bloating and in regulating the energies of the female hormones. Make an oil of the leaves of blessed thistle, the leaves of lavender, and almond oil and massage onto the pelvic area.

- It assists in the healing of pain associated with arthritis. Make a mixture of drops of the essence, a few drops of rose geranium essential oil and almond oil; massage it onto affected areas after bathing.

- It detoxifies the bladder and kidneys. Make an oil from fresh or dried leaves and wheat germ oil and massage the warmed oil onto the kidney and bladder areas after bathing.

- It assists in healing and balancing the heart energy: place plants of blessed thistle around you or take a drop of the essence under your tongue.

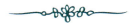

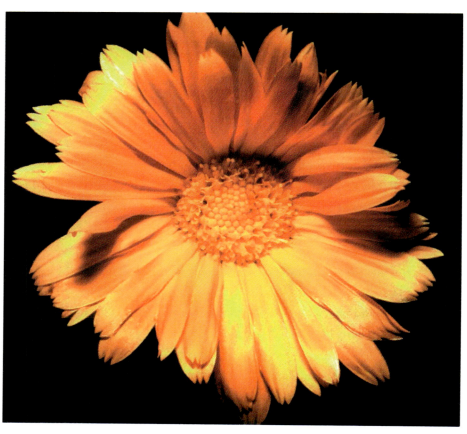

Calendula

Plant Spirit Prayer

*Play with me, oh joyful one, and shine your radiance under the sun.
Bring comfort, joy, and innocence to all, for we behold your
beauty for one so small.*

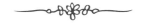

Calendula
(*Calendula officinalis*)

My Experience with This Plant Spirit

In calling on the spirit of the plant, I see an adoring vision of a little girl. She is surrounded by butterflies and kneeling in this enchanted garden of God's creation. She communicates with all of God's creatures, as many are drawn to sitting around this innocent spirit. She is completely joyous and filled with the beauty that surrounds her. The sun shines and radiates its warmth through her very core. Flowering next to her is this vibrant creation of a calendula flower. Its petals are open toward the gentleness of this spirit's face as though to take in her very essence. She becomes smitten at once with the softness and radiance of its colors and leaves and pulls the bloom in close to her to dance upon its magic. The moment she touches it, she also shares with the plant her innocence and jubilation and the two become friends for eternity helping others to heal.

The Spiritual and Emotional Properties

Call on the spirit of this special plant to help children in many ways. It helps them to feel safe in the world when they are all alone. It brings playful childlike energy to all who touch it. It heals the inner child on a deep level. It brings jubilation and joy to one's life. It brings with it a sense of innocence and can help one to create that in their lives. It helps children to laugh, play, and get along better. It comforts little children who might feel alone. It fosters a sense of appropriate sexual energetic boundaries for children who might not have them.

It brings comfort to children whose parents are separated or divorced. It also brings comfort to children when one of the parents is not at home anymore. Call on the spirit of the plant when children are having difficulty with relationships with other kids. It brings life back to children whose souls seem to leave them at a very early age due to some form of abandonment and neglect. It will comfort them and bring them playful spiritual energies to fill their days.

It nurtures an adult's sensual and sexual energy and helps one to feel more attractive within themselves. It will help attract one's soul mate.

The Physical Healing Properties

- Calendula is excellent for tonifying the thymus gland. Make an oil of the leaves of calendula and almond oil and massage the warmed oil over the area of the thymus. Also, placing a drop of the plant spirit essence in water upon waking is helpful.

- It increases sexual energy and libido: place many plants around you and your partner before you retire. Also take 4 drops of the essence in water and sip slowly upon retiring.

- It improves brain function: take a drop of the essence in water when needed. It strengthens heart energy: make a compress of the leaves of calendula and place on top of the chest for fifteen minutes. Do this by moistening the leaves with water and placing them between layers of folded cotton cloth. This is best done in the early evening.

- It is useful for drawing toxins out of the kidneys. Make an oil with wheat germ oil and fresh leaves and flowers and massage the warmed oil onto the kidneys after bathing.

- It helps to alleviate muscle tension. Make a mixture of drops of the essence with olive oil and massage onto muscles after bathing.

- It energetically repels parasites within the digestive tract: place leaves of the plant onto your stomach for twenty-minute intervals. The parasites will be energetically drawn to the calendula and will assist the departure on the physical level.

- It stimulates a sluggish gallbladder. Make an oil with the leaves of the rosemary plant and almond oil. Mix a few drops of calendula essence in the oil and massage onto the gallbladder area.

- It helps to heal the energy around abnormal cell growth in the uterus and cervix. First massage the area with warmed St. John's wort oil. Then make a compress of the flowers and leaves and place on the pubic area for thirty-minute intervals. Do this by moistening the plant parts with warmed almond oil and placing them between layers of folded cotton cloth.

- Calendula is excellent for knee, hip, and other joint injuries. Make an oil of the leaves and flowers with olive oil, then massage onto affected areas after bathing. Do the same for nerve pain in the legs.

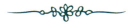

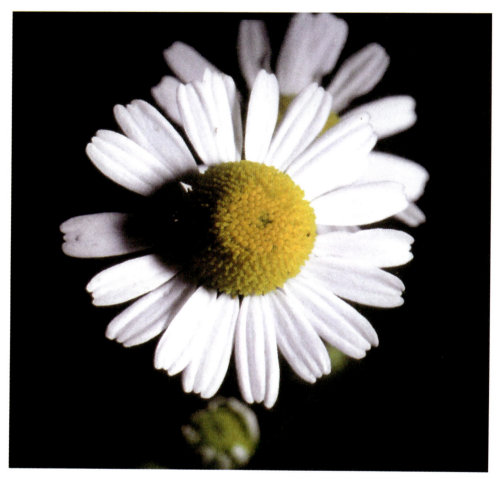

Chamomile

Plant Spirit Prayer

In the angelic whisper of light and love, may we fall upon your wings to shelter us from harm and give us everlasting hope.

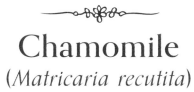

Chamomile
(*Matricaria recutita*)

My Experience with This Plant Spirit

In calling upon the spirit of the plant, a beautiful butterfly comes whispering through the air. Her soft wings flutter aimlessly as she carries herself with the gentlest of ease. The joy of freedom and nonattachment is the gift she bears. And she travels with this from the luminescent clouds to the earth. She is so drawn to the chamomile flower, for she always tends to land on its tiny petals. Being a messenger, she stays for just a short while and carries herself back to the clouds where an angel awaits her return. With open arms and wings of silver, the angel embraces the butterfly and imbues it with angelic healing qualities to bring back to the chamomile plant. Enhanced by the touch of the angel's hand, the butterfly flies away with the magic graced in its wings. Fluttering aimlessly, she dances from flower to flower of each chamomile plant and brings with it the many blessings of the angels above.

The Spiritual and Emotional Properties

Call on the spirit of the plant when there is much confusion. It helps to bring about a sense of calmness and creates space for one to sort things out. Chamomile is very helpful when one is in depression. It works to help heal the emotional energies around alcoholism. It fosters a sense of self-dignity and pride within a person. It is excellent for healing the emotional energies around addictions. It works to balance the emotions and thought patterns. It balances the energy and emotion of unexpressed or overexpressed rage.

It is useful when one is cognizant of dying and helps to foster a sense of inner peace around it. It brings calmness when imminent danger or threat is near.

The Physical Healing Properties

- It works to shift the energy around convulsions: place 10 drops of the essence under the tongue at the onset of the condition.

- It helps to alleviate headaches: take 5–10 drops of the essence in water at the onset of pain.

- It helps calm diarrhea: take 3 drops, three times a day in water until the condition subsides. It helps to calm nausea, vomiting, and tummy ache: make an infusion of the flowers or place drops of the essence in warm water.

- It helps to strengthen the energetic body when one has a virus or influenza. Drink tea made of fresh or dried flowers or place 2 drops of the essence under the tongue upon waking each morning until you begin to feel better.

- It helps to bring nutrients to the bone and helps to maintain bone density in men and women as they age. Taking a few drops of the essence in water daily or drinking a tea made of the flowers is a useful aid for this.

- It soothes diaper rash on a baby's skin. Make an infusion of the fresh flowers in almond oil and massage onto your baby's skin.

- It also helps to heal poison ivy and poison oak. Make an oil of the fresh flowers, St. John's wort flowers or essence, and almond oil, and massage lightly onto affected areas.

- It is a great muscle relaxant. Place a few drops under your tongue when your muscles are feeling a bit stressed!

- For tooth pain, make an infusion of fresh flowers or essence with olive oil and massage onto your gums.

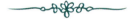

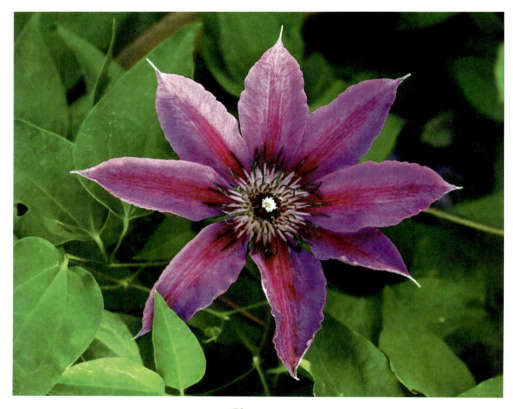

Clematis

Plant Spirit Prayer

We gather here today as your children, the children of the Beloved One Spirit that unites us all. We ask that we be strengthened in your Holy Love and guided to teach the ways of goodness to all peoples of the earth.

Clematis
(Clematis spp.)

My Experience with This Plant Spirit

In calling on the spirit of the plant, a vibrant and colorful woman comes into vision. She is of Indigenous heritage, bearing great strength and wisdom. She is a gatherer of people of all ages and cultures. She stands regally as she calls on those who are called to listen to her message. Many come and sit by her and listen to her words. It is important she shares with us that we all need to take care of each other. No matter who we are or what we look like, we have to respect each other's differences. She says that we must look beyond our appearances and look deep within our hearts. We are all the same, of one God. She gathers the people in closer and asks everyone to join hands. She brings forth a plant of clematis to represent all who have gathered to honor universal love and consciousness. She looks around intently and reminds everyone to love each other as we want to be loved. She makes a blessing over the plant and asks everyone to say their own blessings silently and to send that energy to clematis. It is this powerful union that imbues clematis with its awesome healing abilities.

The Spiritual and Emotional Properties

Call on the spirit of the plant for strength in expressing oneself. It gives those who cannot speak a voice to be heard. It brings healing to self-judgment, self-loathing, and jealousy of others.

Clematis

Clematis brings healing to those who are selfish and self-absorbed, not giving to others or humanity. It heals dishonesty by fostering a conscious awakening in people. For those who push their way through life without regard to others, clematis nudges you to look beyond yourself.

Call on clematis to heal those who are ruthless in their actions. It is the plant of universal love and conscious awakening. It fosters a sense of selflessness in people and creates an environment of sharing. It fosters a sense of community and of reciprocity. It raises the level of consciousness in humanity's ability to give to one another out of love. It also helps to heal hunger, cultural differences, and domestic violence.

The Physical Healing Properties

- Clematis helps to heal the energy around genital herpes: take 4–5 drops of the essence in water upon awakening. One can also place clematis plants next to themselves while they sleep, or soak in a bath imbued with clematis flowers.

- It also helps to heal the herpes-related virus that causes mouth ulcers or canker sores: take a few drops of the essence under your tongue upon waking.

- It helps in the healing of intestinal yeast and fungus: place 1 drop daily under your tongue upon waking. For skin rashes associated with viral infections, make an infusion of the leaves and almond oil and mildly massage onto skin. ***Do not use if there are open sores.***

- For constipation, massage a mixture of warmed wheat germ oil and drops of the essence onto both the pelvis and lower back.

- For worms in the digestive tract, make an infusion of warmed wheat germ oil and leaves of clematis and massage onto the digestive areas.

- It assists in healing the energies surrounding epileptic seizures, dementia, and spasmodic fits. Place many plants around you and call on the spirit for assistance.

- Clematis also has a purifying effect on the blood. Place a drop of the essence in water and take as needed.

- For heavy loss of blood due to miscarriages, place a few drops of the essence in a mixture of almond oil and St. John's wort oil and massage onto pelvis.

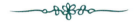

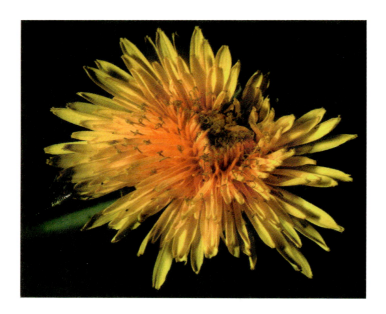

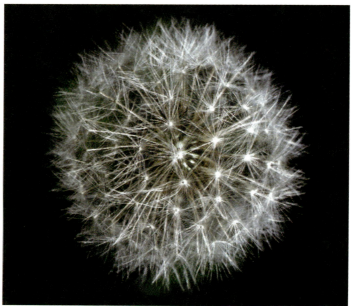

Dandelion

Plant Spirit Prayer

Joyful spirit, full of glee, fill me, embrace me, and shelter me.
Make this magic of most high, grant my dreams unto the sky.

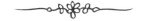

Dandelion
(*Taraxacum officinale*)

My Experience with This Plant Spirit

In calling on the spirit of the plant, your eyes had better be quick to catch this whimsical and magical young lad! It is not hard to find him. For if you look toward the beautiful rainbow in the sky, you will see him sitting with his eyes open wide and a smile as big as the rainbow itself. He is a jovial young boy, and who wouldn't be jovial sitting atop a pot of gold coins amid brilliant colors of light. Lost from his family at birth, he receives joy and healing through creating magic and granting people's wishes. In invoking the spirit of dandelion, this young lad takes one of the gold coins from the pot, brings it to his mouth and blows into it. In the wink of an eye, he becomes surrounded by sparkling fireflies. He turns the gold coin into a magnificent dandelion flower to give to all those who seek to make their wishes come true.

The Spiritual and Emotional Properties

Call on the spirit of the plant when one is faced with depression and inconsolable grief. It assists when one is feeling hopeless from having lost their way in the world. It helps us to be in relationship with the yearning and longing that comes from holding one's integrity as you walk through life's challenges. Dandelion gives you strength as you step into the dark night of the soul only to find the light at the end of the tunnel. It aids in healing the relationship between a mother and daughter. The plant spirit is excellent in working with sudden trauma, loss, or shock. It immediately works to help bring understanding of the situation to one's heart and eases the integration and acceptance process. It assists in reuniting the family structure. Call on dandelion for abundance and good fortune!

The Physical Healing Properties

- Dandelion is a good remedy for healing the energy surrounding hardened arteries. Make a poultice using 2 parts root and 1 part leaf and place on the sternum between the breasts. Do this for twenty-minute intervals, no more than three times per day. Fresh or dried herb can be used.

- To help heal sinus pressure and headache, make a mixture using 12 drops of the essence per tablespoon of olive oil and massage the sinus cavity outward and down toward the neck. Rub also the top of the cervical spine reaching toward the occipital ridge at the base of the cranium.

- For mucous in the lungs, make a mixture of 20 drops of essence in 1/4 cup of warmed wheat germ oil and massage into chest.

- For low blood pressure, rub a few drops of the essence mixed with almond oil onto the wrist pulse points and also on the inside of the foot.

- For poor circulation, mix the essence with almond oil and self-massage daily after bathing.

- For cervical dysplasia (abnormal cell growth in the cervix), make a compress of dried dandelion leaves moistened with warm water in a ratio of 2:1. Take the moistened leaves and place them between layers of folded cotton cloth. Place the compress atop the pubic bone that has first been massaged with warm castor oil for twenty-minute intervals. Late morning to early afternoon is the best time for this.

- For fluid retention from diabetes, make a compress of fresh flowers and warm olive oil to be placed on top of the head for fifteen minutes. Do this by taking the moistened flowers and placing them between layers of folded cotton cloth. When fresh flowers are not available, use 2 tablespoons of warmed castor oil and add 10 drops of the essence and make it into a compress, placing it on the forehead for ten-minute intervals.

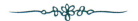

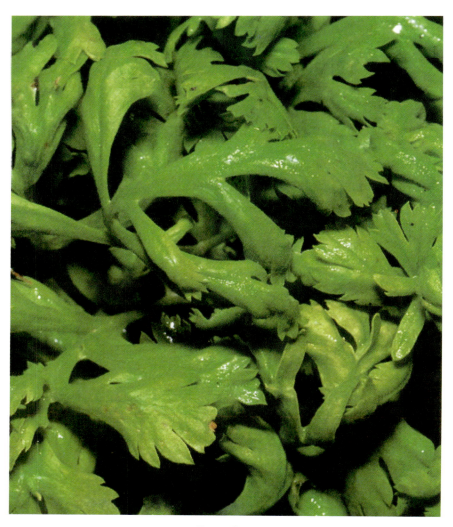

Feverfew

Plant Spirit Prayer

Wanderer of the inner plane, help us to seek that which we yearn to find so deeply within ourselves. Guide us in bringing forth that essence to nurture those we love with it.

Feverfew
(*Tanacetum parthenium*)

My Experience with This Plant Spirit

In calling on the spirit of the plant, a weeping male apparition appears. He carries with him so much sorrow for the life he left behind on earth. He crossed over into the spirit world so suddenly. He has many regrets about not spending enough time with those he loved and also in getting to truly know himself more deeply. His face is withered from emotion and his cloak of pale green is worn from traveling the inner planes in search of one more chance. In his quest to honor himself, he makes a promise to help heal and protect relationships to oneself and others. He travels the ethers to every corner of the world, watching over homes and families and sending healing energies to them. Whenever a family becomes blessed with his healing, a feverfew plant will grow within close proximity to them. When you stumble across feverfew or use it for medicinal purposes, know that the healing energies of relationship are imbued within.

The Spiritual and Emotional Properties

Call on the spirit of the plant to protect one from negative energies and spirits. It assists one in making compromises. It helps one to enjoy life. It heals the energy of male insecurity. It heals the energy of long-held grief and regret. It works to balance pride. Feverfew carries a lot of light. Place it at your door for when loved ones are coming home after a long time away. It holds the sacred space when conflict and healing need to happen. It brings longevity to age.

It keeps honor and integrity at one's place of work. It helps to heal the energy around financial burden. Call on the spirit of feverfew to protect you in the ocean. It assists those who are constantly busy to create time for their families. It helps one to get in touch with their creativity and their feminine aspects of self. It brings artistic culture to one's view of reality.

The Physical Healing Properties

- Feverfew is excellent for healing the energy around nerve pain: take 5 drops of the essence in water upon waking.

- For reducing fevers, make a compress of the leaves and place on the forehead for twenty-minute intervals. Do this by moistening the leaves with a little warmed water and placing them between layers of folded cotton cloth.

- For headaches, place a few drops of the essence in water and sip slowly at the onset of pain.

- For chills, place plants of feverfew around you.

- For throat infections, tonsillitis, and strep throat, make a mixture of drops of the essence, warmed wheat germ oil, and St. John's wort oil and massage onto the throat area.

- For ear infections, make a mixture of drops of the essence and warmed olive oil and massage around the area of the ear and on the outer part of the inside of the ear.

Feverfew 165

- For congestion in the lungs, make an infusion of the leaves and flowers with warmed almond oil and massage onto the chest area.

- To relieve nausea, place a drop of the essence under your tongue. For worms and other toxins in the stomach and digestive tract, take 10–15 drops of the essence in water daily as needed. It balances and tonifies the liver chi: place a few drops of the essence in warmed almond oil and massage onto the liver area.

- Calling on the spirit of the plant and having feverfew around you will help in the following:

    - It assists in healing the energies around learning disabilities.
    - It assists the energy flow for women having uterine contractions and protects the mother as she is about to give birth.
    - It helps to heal the energy around impotence for men.
    - It promotes the energy of fertility and makes the womb and uterus more receptive for communion. It also protects the female during pregnancy when complications arise.

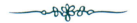

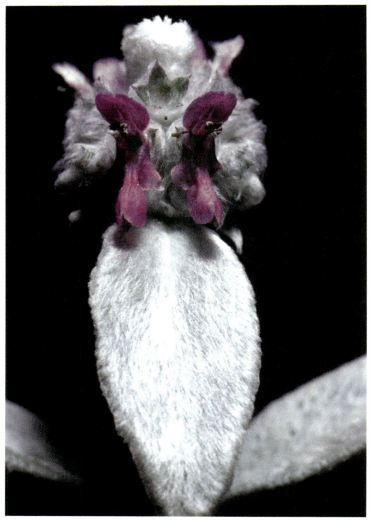

Lamb's Ear

Plant Spirit Prayer

Holy Father, Holy Mother, most powerful of all beings, we call on your Divine assistance to hear our prayers. We ask in thy name to send forth the power of the Holy Spirit to make manifest the miraculous healing abilities of our enlightened ones. We ask this in accordance with the will of God.

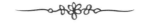

Lamb's Ear
(*Stachys byzantina*)

My Experience with This Plant Spirit

In calling on the spirit of the plant, an elderly male form appears out of the ethers. He is surrounded by penetrating rays of yellow light. His white hair embraces the wrinkles on his tender face, part of which is covered by the beard that he has grown for many years. He wears a modest cloak, for he likes to travel lightly as he has much healing work to do. Every time there is a request for healing from the plant, he makes a journey to answer its prayers. As he nears this sacred shrub, there, protecting it, is a beautiful baby lamb with large and sparkling eyes and a brilliant white coat. He guards the plant and all of the prayers that are made in honor of its name. Every morning, he places his tiny ear next to the leaves and listens to the many requests made for healing. When the time comes for the prayers to be answered, the elderly male spirit nears the lamb and places one of his hands gently over its head and the other over the plant. He imbues the lamb's ear and the animal with holy energy, thus activating its miraculous healing abilities.

The Spiritual and Emotional Properties

Call on the spirit of the plant to help you come to terms with things more peacefully and with less conflict. It is a very special plant. It teaches patience, acceptance, and surrender of what life brings to us. It teaches us how to struggle less and allow for our path to unfold.

The spirit of the plant is used when one feels agitated and frustrated with life. Lamb's ear comforts newborn babies. Place leaves of this plant around very sick children. It will bring them much protection and help for a speedy recovery. The plant spirit also helps one to make peace with things that serve us no longer. It fosters self-love, forgiveness, and aids in the natural process of letting go. It is the plant of surrendering. It brings understanding and peace when one is challenged with major illness. It nourishes our creativity and intuition. It brings back sexual innocence to those who feel they have lost it due to trauma. It helps one to overcome shyness. Call on this plant spirit to help you as you transition from adolescence into puberty and then adulthood.

The Physical Healing Properties

- Lamb's ear is excellent in *energetically* assisting in the healing process around heart attacks, arrhythmia, and strokes: make a large compress by taking the leaves and moistening them with a little warmed water. Place the moistened leaves between folded layers of cotton cloth. Add a few sprigs of violet and place on the chest for twenty-minute intervals; do this as needed.

- It is also helpful in healing the energies around epilepsy and seizure disorders: make a large compress of both fresh leaves of lamb's ear and mullein, moistened with water, and placed on top of the head for an hour. Do this by taking the moistened leaves and placing them between layers of folded cotton cloth.

- For poor eyesight, make a compress of fresh leaves moistened with warm water and place over the eyes for five to seven minutes. This is best done in the morning. For a low-functioning thyroid, take a dosage of 2 drops of the essence in water per day. This is best done upon waking.

- It also is used as a gentle tonifier of the overall endocrine system: take a dosage of 3 drops under the tongue in the early morning. Do this as needed.

- It also tonifies the male reproductive system and prostate glands: take 2–6 drops of essence in water per day.

- Lamb's ear is sacred in that it assists in healing the energies surrounding cancers, such as prostate, esophagus, lung, intestinal, uterine, and cervical cancers. Take 10–20 drops of the essence in water per day. Remember it is important to consult with your health care practitioner when utilizing any alternative methods in conjunction with any treatments you are already using for your illness.

- It is excellent for assisting in the recovery of rape and sexual violence and in the disconnection that might arise in a person from their spirit. Take 1 drop under the tongue in the early morning and massage a mixture of almond oil and drops of the essence onto the pelvic area. See yourself surrounded by blue light and held safely by Spirit.

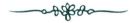

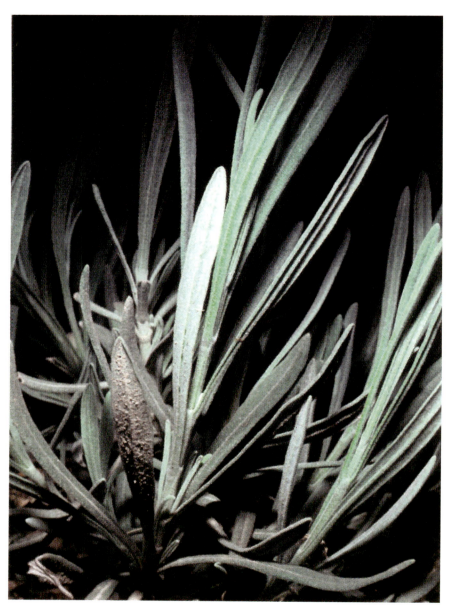

Lavender

Plant Spirit Prayer

Oh, gentle angel with light of spirit, come dance upon me. Wrap your wings around my soul and send unto my heart the light you hold.

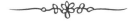

Lavender
(*Lavendula angustifolia*)

My Experience with This Plant Spirit

In calling on the spirit of the plant, a vision of a summer's garden appears to me. A beautiful, young mother is sitting in the sun with her newborn infant cradled in her tender arms. She is nursing her child, feeding her fresh warm milk from her breasts as the sun shines upon the baby's face. They are nestled serenely among plants of lavender. Their gentle fragrance fills the air around them. The mother laughs in utter joy and smiles as she looks down upon her child. The child, receiving the mother's nourishment, coos and grasps tightly onto her mother's nipple for security. The bond between them is so strong and sacred. Being drawn to its hypnotic scent, the mother reaches over to take a sprig of lavender from the plant. She brings it close to her child to smell and then places it in her hair. She watches as her child's face lights up and the two of them become bathed in this effervescent lavender light. The light dances with their every movement and brings to the mother and child energy and grace from the angelic realm. She becomes moved to sit closer to the plant and begins to sing a lullaby in honor and gratitude of the graces bestowed. The plant begins to move gracefully with the melody and align itself with the energies of the mother and child. It is this song that activates the healing properties of the lavender plant. Whenever you stumble across some lavender, look to see if it is dancing. You just might hear its lullaby!

The Spiritual and Emotional Properties

Call on the spirit of the plant when you are healing from a broken heart. It brings happiness when there is misery. Put sprigs of lavender around you to attract your life partner. It will bring you good fortune. Lavender brings life and light to your heart. It is healing in that it creates laughter and cheer. Call on the plant spirit to bring joy to babies and children.

It aligns the heart chakras of partners for eternity. It is nourishing for one's energy field and brings in with it a higher vibration of spiritual energy. Placing lavender plants around you will help you to communicate with your deceased loved ones. Beings who have crossed over use lavender as a doorway into this reality and are drawn by its fragrant smell. It is an excellent tool in healing rips and tears in the energy field. It helps to heal unresolved karmic issues and past incarnations.

The Physical Healing Properties

- Lavender is excellent for tonifying the lymphatic system: take 2 drops of the essence in water per day.

- It is helpful for soothing sinus inflammation. Add a few drops of the essence in warmed olive oil and massage onto inflamed areas.

- Lavender also assists in the healing of a mild burn. Forty-eight hours after receiving the burn, crush fresh lavender flowers and infuse them into a mixture of 1 part almond oil and 2 parts grape-seed oil. Massage lightly onto affected areas.

- It is helpful in healing intestinal yeast, or a rash due to fungal infection, and other rashes due to dampness and mold exposure: take 3 drops of the essence per day under tongue as needed.

- Lavender strengthens the kidneys, adrenal glands, and liver. Make

Lavender 173

a mixture of the essence mixed with jojoba oil and massage over the intended areas.

- For regulating the spleen and pancreas, make an oil with almond oil, fresh violet flowers, and drops of the essence, add a touch of honey, and massage onto the spleen and pancreas.

- It is useful in alleviating the discomfort of indigestion: make a compress of fresh or dried flowers, and fresh or dried rosemary herb, and place on stomach for ten to fifteen minutes. Do this by taking the herb and moistening with warmed water and then placing the plant parts between layers of folded cotton cloth. Before laying the compress, massage the area with warmed olive oil.

- To alleviate menstrual bloating, massage a mixture of drops of the essence and jojoba oil onto the pelvic area. It is also useful in healing vaginal yeast infections: make a compress using fresh or dried herb, moistened with warm water, and place over pubic bone for twenty minutes. Do this by placing the herb between layers of folded cotton cloth. It is beneficial to first massage the area with warmed St. John's wort oil.

- For bladder infections and toxicity in the bladder, make a compress of fresh or dried herb and place over pubic bone for twenty-minute intervals. Do this by moistening the herb with a little water and placing it between layers of folded cotton cloth. First massage the area with warmed wheat germ oil. Placing a heating pad over the compress increases the healing effect.

- For eye strain and discomfort, make a compress using just fresh lavender leaves and place it on top of the eyes for ten-minute intervals.

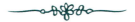

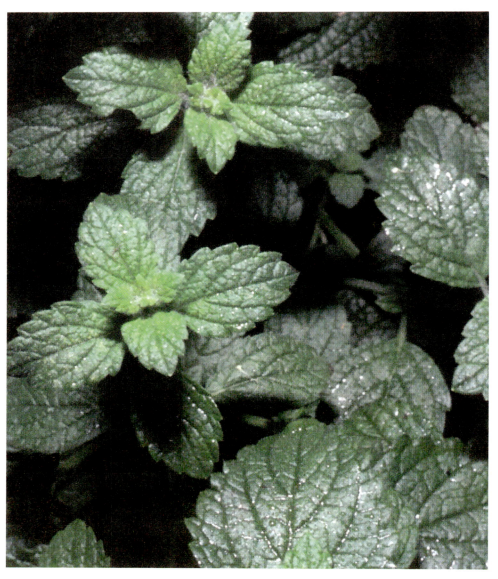

Lemon Balm

Plant Spirit Prayer

Fly little fairy as fast as you can and bring magic to each lemon balm with the stroke of your hand. Using your wand filled with God's grace, make nectar of its leaves for the entire human race.

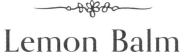

Lemon Balm
(*Melissa officinales*)

My Experience with This Plant Spirit

In calling on the spirit of the plant, a tiny effervescent fairy comes whizzing by me. She is a delicate and strong-willed spirit, and she carries with her a wand of magic. She stands guard over the lemon balm plant and has many messengers to help her in her venture. One of them is the royal queen bee. This bee travels from leaf to leaf listening to the healing wishes of those who seek its medicine. Upon hearing the messages, the bee calls for the fairy's assistance. This flamboyant spirit manifests its presence and sets itself upon each leaf. By virtue of tapping its magic wand, the healing properties of lemon balm become activated.

The Spiritual and Emotional Properties

Call on the spirit of lemon balm to help you overcome the fear of being in the world and walking in your own shoes. Lemon balm gives you that courage. It helps to heal injustice. It helps those who believe that life is unfair to see the broader picture. It gives one strength to work through unjust and unfair treatment. When a part of a person's lifeforce is taken from them in a situation, the spirit of lemon balm will help to soothe that soul. It helps one to maintain mental and emotional strength. It also overcomes fatigue associated with mental and emotional challenges. It gives one the strength to persevere when fighting for a good cause. It assists in healing the energy around heartache.

It helps the givers in life learn to receive as well. Call on the spirit of lemon balm when you are making amends with your children. It is the plant of gathering for spiritual communion. It helps one aspire to the spiritual life.

The Physical Healing Properties

- Lemon balm is excellent for healing the energetic effects of smoking in the lungs: take 4 drops of the plant spirit essence in water a few times a day.

- For lung congestion and phlegm associated with bronchitis, pneumonia, and coughs, take 10–20 drops of the essence in water a few times a day and also massage a mixture of drops of the essence and warmed wheat germ oil over the lung area.

- For head congestion, inflammation in sinus membranes, and ear congestion, add drops of the essence to your bathwater. Also make an oil with the fresh or dried flowers and apricot kernel oil and massage around various areas of the head and face.

- For phlegm in the throat, make a mixture of olive oil, St. John's wort oil, and drops of the essence and massage onto throat area.

- Lemon balm acts as a cooling agent when there is too much heat in the digestive system: place drops of the essence in almond oil and massage onto stomach.

- It also is an excellent stress alleviator and helps one to feel calmer: place a drop of the essence under your tongue when feeling a little overwhelmed.

- It stimulates the flow of the intestines and rectum and therefore assists in relieving constipation: make a mixture of drops of the essence and warmed olive oil and massage onto your lower back after bathing.

- It is helpful for stimulating kidney and adrenal function: make a mixture of almond oil and drops of the essence and massage onto your kidney and adrenal area.

- It brings physical and mental stamina and helps to alleviate fatigue: place a few drops of the essence under your tongue or have lots of lemon balm plants around your home.

- It relieves muscle spasms in the uterine area: make a mixture of almond oil, St. John's wort oil, and drops of the essence and massage onto the affected area.

- It increases overall circulation: add drops of the essence to your bathwater; or make an infusion of the flowers, and drink.

- It is excellent in working with allergies that arise from airborne organisms. Drink a tea made from an infusion of the flowers or take drops of the essence under the tongue upon waking.

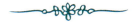

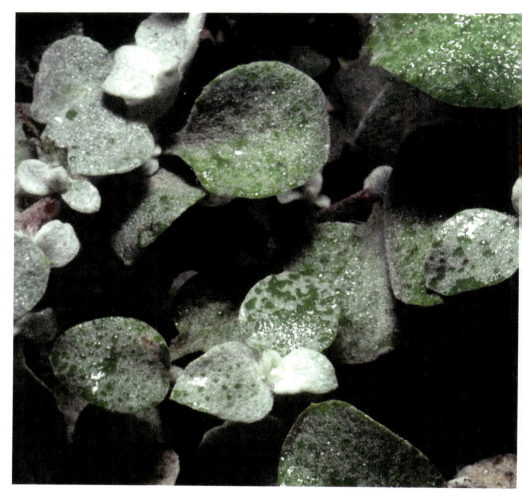

Licorice

Plant Spirit Prayer

Harmony of spirit, harmony of creation . . . performed by the hands of greatness and instilled in splendor. Heal us with thy sounds and create the space for hope, healing, and God to manifest in all.

Licorice
(*Glycyrrhiza glabra*)

My Experience with This Plant Spirit

In calling on the spirit of the plant, a great being appears before me. He is a very easygoing spirit. He carries with him an old guitar whose strings are worn and tired with age. He has played music with it since his time on earth and took it with him when he crossed over. His life was a very poor one. He went around mostly with the clothes on his back and ate what food was given to him, only you wouldn't know it by the demeanor on his face. His music kept alive his faith in God and in humanity. He never stopped trusting even though at times he wasn't supported in his physical existence. He always said that was ok with him; he trusted in the land and that God took care of him always. He would take long walks in the woods and on the beaches and strum his guitar as he lay on the ground. Many times, he would unintentionally lie near a licorice plant. Over time, he formed a special bond with these plants and would strum his guitar every time he came upon one. The plants took a fancy to him too. They would light up every time he came by. When the time came for him to leave the earth, they were very saddened and hoped to stay connected. One day, music from the sky came down upon the plants, and they recognized the strum of those old guitar strings.

Their old friend had returned and continues to imbue the licorice plants with their magical healing qualities.

The Spiritual and Emotional Properties

Call on the spirit of the plant to heal those who have been emotionally and physically wounded in wars. It brings peace to war veterans who have suffered physical loss. It brings comfort and nurturing to those who have no family, and to those who are outcasts of society. It brings peace to those who are suffering from devastating illnesses, which our society looks down upon. It helps to heal the energies surrounding a difficult child labor and birthing. It heals the energies of societal and cultural issues. Call on the spirit of the plant to heal the hearts of the despondent of our society, the poor, and the suppressed. It heals the spiritual energies around present day slavery in third world countries and others as well. In prisons, it fosters the energy of hope, support, and transformation for those who want to turn their lives around. It heals the karmic energy of all societal abuses. It also heals the energies around grievances in past lives and offers resolution.

The Physical Healing Properties

- Licorice is an excellent energy booster to the body: place a few drops of the plant spirit essence under your tongue.

- For breathing difficulties and asthma, take 4 drops of the essence in water upon waking. Also massage a mixture of drops of the essence and warmed olive oil onto your chest after bathing.

- It stimulates the kidneys and adrenals: make a mixture of drops of the essence and almond oil and massage onto the area after bathing.

- It clears inflammation of the sinuses, lungs, and breathing passages: place 10 drops of the essence in warmed water and sip slowly. Also make an oil with the leaves of licorice and warmed olive oil and massage onto the chest and sinus area before retiring.

- It stimulates digestion and the liver. Massage a mixture of drops of the essence and avocado oil onto those areas before retiring.

- It helps with morning sickness: place 2 drops of the essence in warm water and drink in the morning.

- It is helpful for removing bladder toxicity: make a compress of the leaves of licorice and place on top of the bladder area for twenty-minute intervals. Do this by taking the leaves and moistening them with a little warmed water and placing them between folded layers of cotton cloth. It is beneficial to massage the area first with a little warmed almond oil and then place a heating pack on top of the compress. This is best done in the early evening.

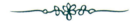

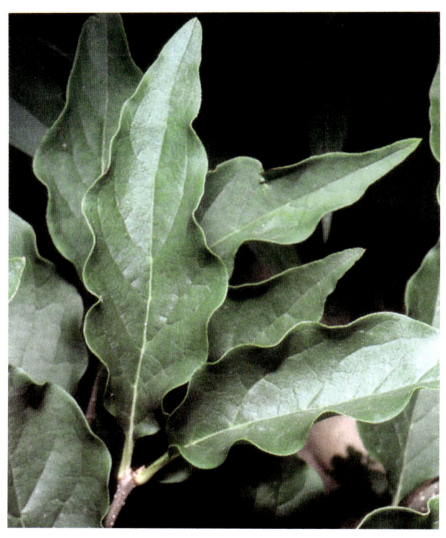

Lilac

Plant Spirit Prayer

Oh love, pure love, be still my heart. Nourish it with everlasting bliss and blessings of most high. Bring forth union of body, of mind, of spirit, of myself, and with another. I place my soul within the gentleness of your tiny petals and entrust the well-being of my heart's journey in your graces.

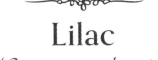

Lilac
(*Syringa vulgaris*)

My Experience with This Plant Spirit

In calling on the spirit of the plant, a beautiful young woman of innocence, dressed in shimmering white, appears to me. With her arms dancing with subtle movements of grace, she moves her feet in harmony to the gentle sounds of the wind. She saunters around the lilac bush, enchantingly picking its flowers. Her dress flowing and catching on branches, she is completely filled with joy and contentment. She is to be joined in spiritual union with another, and this so fills her being with radiant love. This love penetrates so powerfully from her heart that it touches each and every lilac flower as she dances by it. She imbues the lilac with grace, serenity, and everlasting content, and blesses all those who call on the plant for assistance. From henceforth, all unions of body, mind, spirit—to oneself and one another—shall have the special blessing of the lilac bush.

The Spiritual and Emotional Properties

Call on the spirit of this wonderful plant when one is transitioning through life. Lilac is symbolic of transition. It assists a woman energetically as she transitions through menopause. This special time in a woman's life should be blessed by the lilac bush, as it helps in the integration and changes that take place in a woman physically, emotionally, and spiritually. Call on lilac when you are missing someone. It helps to soothe one's heart. It brings comfort to the grieving process when one has just lost their life partner in death. Lilac is the flower of romance. Call on the plant spirit to help bring romance back into a relationship or to help find some. It is wonderful in assisting you in attracting that special someone to your life. The lilac bush honors rites of passage for both men and women. It has a special relationship to grandparents and the spirit of the plant can be called upon in healing those relationships. It blesses wedding days and marriages and brings luck to the bride and groom. It honors sacred union between two people and helps to rekindle that energy. It also blesses friendship. It can also be called upon to communicate with your animals and calm them when they are in distress. The lilac flower brings much contentment and fulfillment.

The Physical Healing Properties

- Lilac is excellent for healing the energies around pneumonia, bronchitis, and chest colds. Make an oil of fresh or dried flowers, with equal parts warmed almond and olive oils and massage onto chest.

- For loss of circulation in extremities, mix a few drops of the essence with olive oil and massage.

- To bring warmth to the body when it is cold, take a few drops of essence under your tongue. It also improves circulation in the lymphatic system. Add a few drops of the essence into warmed wheat germ oil and massage onto your body.

- For energetically dispersing candida and intestinal yeast, take 10–15 drops of essence daily under the tongue.

- It aids in detoxifying and tonifying the gallbladder: make a compress using fresh or dried flowers and place on gallbladder area for twenty minutes. Do this by moistening the leaves with a little warmed wheat germ oil and placing them between layers of folded cotton cloth.

- It also helps to tonify and detoxify the kidneys: make an oil with almond oil and fresh or dried flowers and massage onto the kidney area.

- It helps with heavy menses: massage onto pelvic area a mixture of almond oil with a few drops of the essence.

- Lilac is an excellent hormone regulator. It helps to alleviate some of the symptoms associated with menopause such as irritability, mood swings, and hot flashes: take 8–10 drops of the essence in water, one to three times a day. Tune in to the amount and dosage you need. Each woman's body and energy system are different and call for varying amounts. Always start out once a day and see how your body works with the lilac essence.

- For a vaginal yeast infection, take 3 drops of essence three times a day under the tongue.

- It also assists in regulating the functions of the pancreas: make a compress of fresh or dried flowers moistened with olive oil and place over pancreas for ten minutes. Do this by taking the moistened flowers and placing them between layers of folded cotton cloth. When fresh or dried flowers are not available, use the essence. This will assist in healing the energy surrounding blood sugar imbalances.

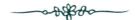

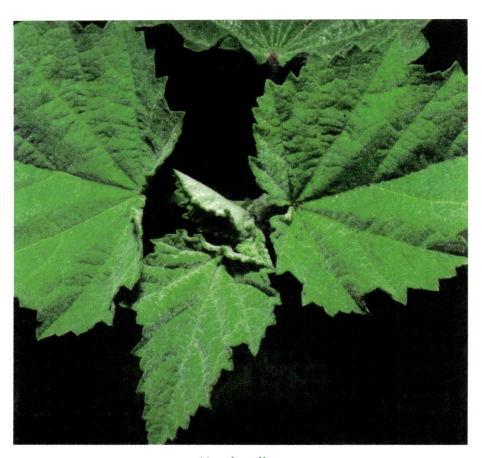

Marshmallow

Plant Spirit Prayer

Divine Will, assist me in harnessing the innate power of my true and authentic self. Help hold in my vision, my destiny, and give me the courage to manifest it in physical reality.

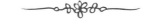

Marshmallow
(*Althea officinalis*)

My Experience with This Plant Spirit

In calling on the spirit of the plant, many sages and mystics appear to me from the ethers. They spend their time delegating and watching over the paths and journeys of human beings. They gently offer guidance and assistance when needed, subtly working with the spiritual energies surrounding a person's destiny. They often help us when we tend to get ourselves in the way of the highest good unfolding for us. They usually do this without our knowing, as they are our secret spiritual helpers. Every time they assist one of us, they grow a marshmallow plant on the earth to remind us to keep aligned with the will of our highest selves. When one uses the plant for healing purposes, they are also receiving the energies of the miraculous endeavors of these sages and mystics of old.

The Spiritual and Emotional Properties

Call on the spirit of the plant when one is feeling overwhelmed by their circumstances and not able to control what is happening in their lives. It will bring much ease, comfort, and understanding of the energy unfolding. It is good for protection against negative energies and influences. When one can't figure out things, marshmallow is excellent for working through confusion to find out what makes sense. When one has lost their sense of physical direction, marshmallow will help you to get where you need to go. Call on the spirit of the plant to help heal regrets. It is also helpful in healing the souls of those spirits who are still wandering the ethers with many regrets in their hearts. Marshmallow is excellent for helping one to create structure and balance in their lives. When one has to ground an idea into physical reality, marshmallow holds the space for that and fosters motivation and personal will. It gives one energy to complete tasks. It fosters a sense of authority, a sense of personal purpose and power. Call on the spirit of marshmallow to help you fulfill your soul's destiny.

The Physical Healing Properties

- Marshmallow tonifies and strengthens the digestive system and stomach chi: take 4 drops of the plant spirit essence in water upon waking.

- It is also good for strengthening the colon and for relieving the inflammation of hemorrhoids: steep the leaves of marshmallow in warmed olive oil for an hour or so, and massage on the lower part of the back and around the rectal area.

- It improves circulation: mix drops of the essence with almond oil and massage onto body after bathing.

- It improves brain function and brings clarity to one's mental state: place plants of marshmallow around you and place a drop of the essence under the tongue upon retiring.

- It works to energetically clear and dispel parasites and worms in the digestive tract: place a few drops of the essence in warmed water and drink as a tea before retiring. Also make a compress with the leaves of marshmallow and place on the stomach for twenty-minute intervals. Do this by taking the leaves and moistening them with a little warmed water and placing them between layers of folded cotton cloth. This is best done in the early evening before eating a large meal.

- It is excellent in assisting the healing of some types of skin rashes, wounds, and sores. Make an oil of the leaves of marshmallow, flowers of lemon balm, and almond oil. Massage onto the skin as needed. ***Do not use on open wounds or sores that are bleeding.***

- It is a good cleanser for the gallbladder. Massage the area first with warmed wheat germ oil, then make a compress using the leaves and place on the gallbladder area for twenty minutes. Do this by taking the leaves, moistening them with a little warmed water and placing them between layers of folded cotton cloth.

- When blood sugar levels are too high, marshmallow helps to bring them down by balancing the energies of the spleen and pancreas. Make a mixture of drops of the essence in warmed olive oil and massage onto the area of the spleen and pancreas.

- It is a good remedy for healing ulcers: make a mixture using warmed olive oil, apricot kernel oil, drops of marshmallow essence, and a few drops of the lavender essence. Massage onto the stomach area after bathing.

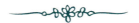

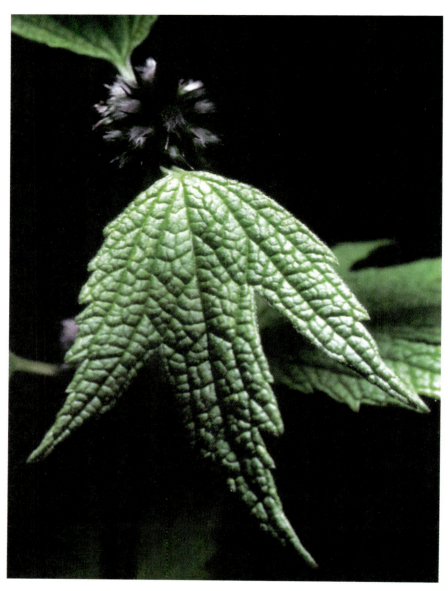

Motherwort

Plant Spirit Prayer

Rejoice, oh noble one! For the kingdom of heaven is upon us.
In your glory, may miracles of God abound everywhere.

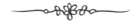

Motherwort
(*Leonurus cardiaca*)

My Experience with This Plant Spirit

In calling on the spirit of the plant, a vision appears of many spirits playing their trumpets as they wait for a special being to join them. They announce her entrance with the songs of the heavens, and upon their last note, a regal being appears with all her glory. She is a queen in the spirit world. She knows exactly what her purpose and mission is and is ready and willing to perform her duties. As the trumpets continue to blare, she raises her hands and delegates to all those who serve her and perform their duties on behalf of human consciousness. She works in the energetic field of human evolution, in the spiritual dimensions creating many miracles on a daily basis. She doesn't wait to be asked for help. She sees where her assistance is needed and facilitates a healing. Every time she does this, she grows a motherwort plant on the earth plane. When one uses the plant for medicinal purposes, know that you are receiving the energy of the miracle that was performed by this noble spirit!

The Spiritual and Emotional Properties

Motherwort is a protector of the soul force of humanity. Call on the spirit of the plant to nurture the family unit as a whole as it brings grace to the family. It protects babies in the spirit world as they are ready to incarnate into the physical reality. It acts as a guide and directs the spirit. It holds space for the soul's evolutionary growth. It heals the spirits of abandoned children, children who are lost to drugs, violence, and abuse. Call on the spirit of the plant to heal the spirits around those who are homeless. It bestows graces upon humanity and gives direction to one's life. It will help keep you on your path, aligned with God, and will continue to guide you through life.

Physical Healing Properties

- Motherwort is a very powerful spiritual healing plant. It is used to heal the energies that surround many autoimmune illnesses that affect brain and nervous system functioning.

- It heals the energies around Lou Gehrig's disease, and Parkinson's disease.

- It heals the energies surrounding brain aneurysms: call on the spirit of motherwort to assist you with those, place many plants around you, and also take a few drops of the essence in water upon waking.

- It is excellent in healing the energy around a heart attack and stroke: placing plants around you is a wonderful remedy, and also placing 2 drops of the essence under your tongue upon retiring. Placing a compress of the leaves of motherwort on the heart area will also help to heal the energy. Moisten the leaves with a little warmed water and fold it between layers of cotton cloth. Gently place on the heart area for twenty-minute intervals. This is best done in the evening.

- It heals the energies around tumors of the liver, spleen, pancreas, lymphatic system, intestines, and colon. Make an oil with the leaves in olive oil and St. John's wort oil and massage the warmed oil over the affected areas.

- It works to heal the energy around stomach ulcers and ailments: make a compress of leaves of motherwort moistened with a generous amount of warmed almond oil and place on the stomach area for fifteen-minute intervals. Do this by placing the moistened leaves between layers of folded cotton cloth. Adding direct heat by use of a heating pad would be very beneficial.

- It is also helpful in healing the energetic trauma from injuries to the physical body that directly relates to the spine. Make an oil of the leaves, almond oil, and St. John's wort oil and massage onto the spine; do this after bathing.

- It also induces rest. Take a few drops of the essence in water upon retiring and sip slowly. When one is undergoing major surgery, call on the spirit of motherwort to protect and heal you.

- It works to heal the scar tissue that manifests in the energy field after surgery. Make an oil with a few drops of the essence and olive oil and massage directly onto the mature scar tissue.

- It heals the energy around a heart murmur: massage a little almond oil with a few drops of the essence added directly onto the heart and chest area.

- To heal the energy around muscle apathy, massage a mixture of drops of the essence in almond oil onto the body after bathing.

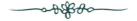

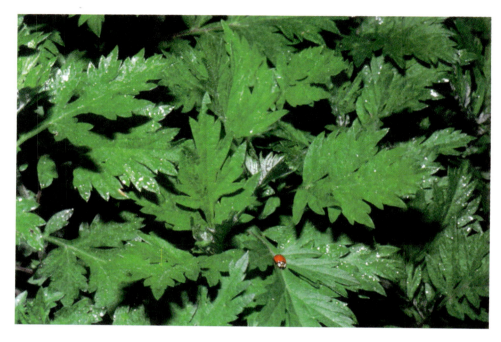

Mugwort

Plant Spirit Prayer

*We call on you, ancestors of the earth and sky.
Hear our prayers. We need your medicine to heal our people
and Mother Earth. We thirst for wholeness. We hunger for nourishment.
Carry us in your womb as we walk this earth. Protect us from harm.
Feed our children. And when we are ready to come home to the
Great Spirit in the sky, carry us on your wings and fly!*

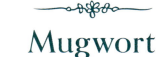

Mugwort
(*Artemesia vulgaris*)

My Experience with This Plant Spirit

In calling on the spirit of the plant, a medicine man comes toward me and sits in the dirt around a blazing fire. He is chanting while holding a piece of mugwort plant cupped in his hands. He rocks back and forth over the fire, drawing the plant to his mouth and forehead, each time saying a prayer for the earth. He then takes his hand and circles the fire. This is to symbolize the cycle of life, of birth to death, of completion. He invokes special prayers into the plant and calls on the ancestors of the earth and sky to help instill power for the medicinal and spiritual healing properties. He makes an offering and places the mugwort into the fire as a gifting for the healing of humanity.

The Spiritual and Emotional Properties

Call on the spirit of the plant to walk with you hand to hand in life. It is used to foster motivation in oneself and helps to create the desire needed to live on the earth plane. It helps to increase sexual desire toward one's partner. The plant spirit is excellent for healing from issues of sexual trauma. It helps to make whole and to gently integrate the soul pieces during recovery. It works with healing the trauma suffered from violence. Call on this plant spirit when you have suffered physical injury. It also helps in the recovery of alcoholic abuse by helping the substance user to gather strength in working through their issues.

Mugwort is used to cross over into the spirit world. It is the plant of journeying. Call on mugwort to heal other spirits who are lost and still wandering in other dimensional realities. It helps them to find their way back home. It is used for spiritual protection and for clearing negative energies from one's energy field. The plant spirit aids in a safe journey when one is in the dying process. It is also called upon for bringing in good harvest and protecting the children. It is a very powerful spiritual plant.

The Physical Healing Properties

- Mugwort is excellent for clearing energetic mucous from the body: place a few drops of the essence in water and drink upon waking.

- For dryness of the mouth, lungs, and chest, make a mixture of drops of the essence and warmed almond oil and massage onto the chest and lung area.

- For fluid in the ears from colds and sinus problems, place 2 drops of the essence in 1 tablespoon of warmed olive oil and place in the ears.

- For indigestion and weak digestion, first massage that area with warmed avocado oil, then take fresh leaves and place it on the stomach for an hour.

- For sore eyes due to allergies, make a compress using the leaves and place it on the eyes for ten-minute intervals. Do this by moistening the leaves with a little warmed water and placing them between layers of folded cotton cloth.

- For fluid retention associated with urinary tract infections and incontinence, massage castor oil onto the lower abdominal region and place fresh leaves on top. When fresh leaves are not available, make a compress using the dried herb moistened with olive oil.

- For stiffness in the joints, lower back pain, and kidney discomfort, combine olive oil with a generous dosage of the essence, and massage the warmed oil onto the affected areas.

- For menstrual discomfort, make an infusion of equal parts olive oil and fresh or dried herb, and a tablespoon of crushed rosemary, and massage it into the pelvis area.

- For minor cuts, scrapes, and mosquito bites, make a paste using equal parts of crushed fresh or dried herb and olive oil, and 1/2 teaspoon of bentonite clay, and place on the affected area. ***Do not use on open wounds***.

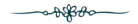

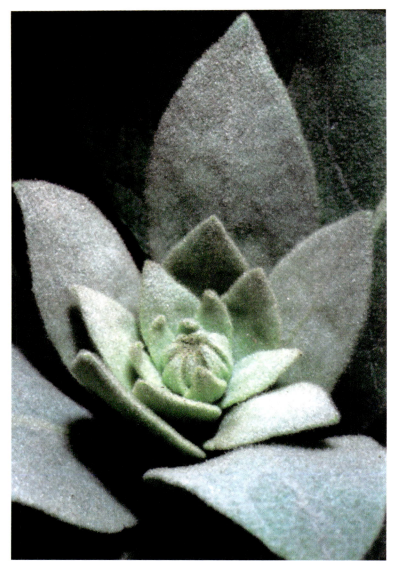

Mullein

Plant Spirit Prayer

Oh, gentleness, oh wonder, oh God's creation, bring forth your sunshine, your ray of hope. Manifest through the glory of God your eternal presence and unto us, shine in the light of angel's wings.

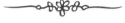

Mullein
(*Verbascum thapsus*)

My Experience with This Plant Spirit

In calling on the spirit of the plant, a gentle female voice comes to me. She has no form, for she is just light. The energy around her voice is one of mystery and hurriedness; for this plant spirit is very busy being caretaker of the plant kingdom. She tells me she is the keeper of the mullein plant, the protectorate of its life-force. She watches over all of Mother Earth, our Garden of Eden. She brings sunshine and creates harmony within the plant world. She travels from one plant to the other, spreading her nourishment. When I asked this plant spirit for assistance, she answered my call and appeared in the form of a ladybug sitting atop a mullein leaf. She does not draw attention to herself . . . she comes to bring her medicine and quickly goes on her way to where she is needed next.

The Spiritual and Emotional Properties

Call on this plant spirit for support and encouragement. It is helpful when one is in a constant state of worry or is overwhelmed. When you think you can't make it through the day, the spirit will help to alleviate your stress. The plant spirit heals strife and conflict within the family unit. It also helps to bring forgiveness when there is anger. Call on the spirit of mullein when your loved ones are missing or little children wander off and become lost. It helps to honor the connection when loved ones are far away or separated. It helps to combat boredom and fosters excitement. It also helps one to feel safe in this world.

It is called upon for increasing one's connection and faith in a higher power. It brings magic and surprises to one's life. It helps in maintaining a healthy connection between a person's lower and higher selves. It keeps you aligned with Spirit.

The Physical Healing Properties

- Mullein is excellent for healing the energies around asthma, lung infections, bronchitis, and shallow breathing: take 20–30 drops of the essence in water per day.

- For lethargy, place the plant near you at night when you sleep.

- For healing the energy around multiple sclerosis, drink a tea made from an infusion of the leaves.

- For weakness in the legs, make a mixture of drops of the essence and rosemary oil and massage onto the legs.

- For emphysema, take 10 drops of the essence per day and massage an oil of crushed leaves and warmed olive oil onto the chest.

- For baby's diaper rash, massage a few drops of the essence mixed with olive oil.

- For prickly heat and other inflamed rashes, make a paste of fresh crushed mullein leaves, crushed juniper berries, and olive oil and place the mixture on the rash for twenty-minute intervals a few times per day.

- For mercury and chemical toxicity, kidney toxicity, and environmental toxins in the body, drink an infusion of the leaves.

- For burning skin from environmental pollutants, mix the essence with almond oil and massage generously into the skin.

- For eczema, psoriasis, and other skin rashes due to digestive disturbances, make a paste using bentonite clay, mullein leaves, and olive oil and place on the skin for ten to fifteen minutes once a day.

- For arthritis, make the same paste as above and leave on the inflamed area for an hour wrapped in cotton cloth. This is best done in the evening before retiring.

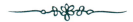

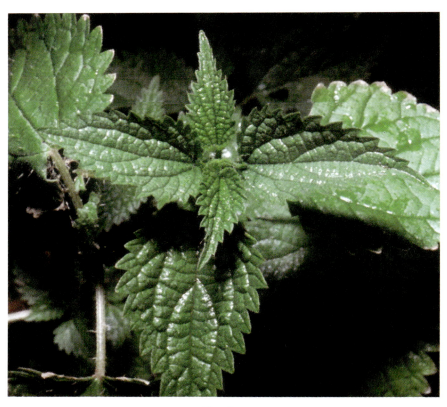

Nettles

Plant Spirit Prayer

Oh, Loving Kindness, drench the fires of our bitterness and scorn.
Weep not, for the ills of the human heart can only be appeased
by that of your unbounded gracious love.

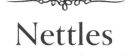

Nettles
(*Urtica dioica*)

My Experience with This Plant Spirit

In calling upon the spirit of the plant, I saw not one, but two spirits hiding among the leaves. They are the fairies of this wondrous plant, and their arms were swinging in motion to the rhythm of their stinging tails that follow along behind them. One fairy is male and the other is female. He is the bitter of the two. His feelings of being unwanted and unloved permeate from his being. He is angry at the world, refusing to believe in goodness and loving kindness. He sits upon the leaves and instills his scorn into the plant to make it as unlovable as he.

The other fairy is the one who holds the light for the nettles plant. She is a gentle being, loving, compassionate, and trusting of the world. She will stay with nettles and imbue it with love as long as the other is there. She will radiate loving kindness to the plant to help keep the energies in balance with each other. She keeps her heart open toward the other fairy, constantly sending him unconditional love and acceptance. It is this balance of the two that gives the nettles plant its wondrous healing abilities.

The Spiritual and Emotional Properties

Call on the spirit of the plant to assist you when you are thinking negative thoughts. It helps when you are feeling negative emotions that aren't serving your highest good. Nettles helps to heal the energy around bitterness and scorn. It dissipates vengeful thoughts when one is having them toward another. It works to heal jealousy and envy. It helps to bring one out of the state of selfishness and self-absorption. It fosters empathy for others. Nettles is excellent in working with those who are possessive, obsessive, and controlling. Nettles will bring a change of heart in a person. It is excellent for grounding and will align your source of power with that of Divine Right. It is useful in bringing some resolution in marital conflict and divorce.

The Physical Healing Properties

- Nettles is excellent for sinus and lung congestion due to allergens by helping to build up the immune system's natural defenses. Take 5 drops of the essence under the tongue upon waking.

- For bronchitis, make a mixture of the essence and warmed wheat germ oil and massage onto the chest area upon retiring.

- To help energetically clear the lymphatic system, take 3–6 drops of the essence in water two to three times a day.

- Nettles is an overall blood strengthener and builder: drink a tea of the leaves or place 5–7 drops of the essence in warm water. It is excellent for anemia and replenishing iron. One can make a tea of the leaves for this as well or place a few drops of the essence under the tongue upon waking.

- When a female is heavily menstruating, nettles help with the loss of minerals from the blood. Taking 10–15 drops of the essence while menstruating is a good remedy for this.

- It also helps to alleviate stomach acid and works to calm digestive problems. Make a mixture of the essence and almond oil and massage onto the stomach after bathing.

- It is good for strengthening the liver: make a mixture of the essence and wheat germ oil and massage onto the liver area.

- It cleanses the gallbladder and stomach: drink a tea of the fresh leaves before retiring.

- Nettles will help heal the energy around arthritis: take 5–10 drops of the essence in water per day upon waking.

- It cleanses the intestines and colon: take dried leaves and simmer (covered) for 20 minutes, and slowly sip the tea in the evening time.

- It also builds strength in the body: place a drop of the essence under your tongue when you are feeling fatigued.

- The nettles plant has stinging hairs on each leaf. When collecting the plant, it is advisable to use gloves unless it is collected very early in the spring. When brewing the leaves to make a tea, the stingers become deactivated.

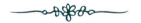

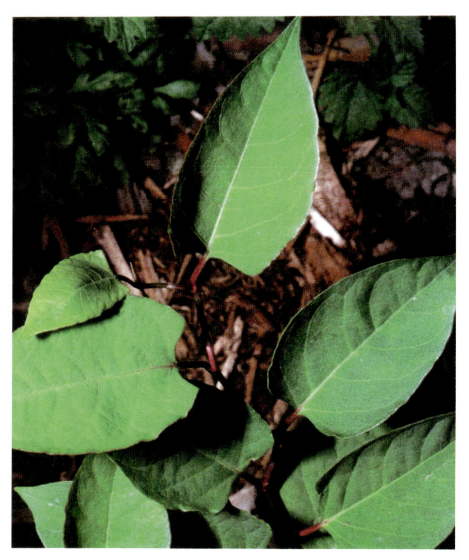

Poke

Plant Spirit Prayer

Great Creator and Spirit of the buffalo, we surrender to your powerful medicine. We stand here before you, seeking guidance and direction. Bring to us your wisdom, great spirits, so that we may follow in the trails you leave behind. Show us the way, for we are your children.

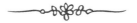

Poke
(*Phytolacca americana*)

My Experience with This Plant Spirit

In calling on the spirit of the plant, a beautiful dark-skinned Native woman comes forth. She is adorned with leather buffalo hides and intricate beadwork in colors of blue and pink. Her hands are outstretched as if to embrace the mysteries of life. Surrounding her are flames of red fire bursting from the earth, crying out for the wounds of humanity. She calls out to white buffalo. There, appearing before her is a sacred white buffalo of enormous stature and presence. With markings of deep red painted over its body, they symbolize the sufferings of the mother. This magnificent creature brings with it all the medicines necessary for healing the spirit of the earth's people. It angrily prances around setting its hoofs upon the flames, giving over to the fire the anger of the human race for purification.

After sharing its wisdom received from the ritual, the buffalo leaves to return to its source, leaving behind a powerful poke plant. The Native woman sits near the plant and makes an offering of a strand of her hair and thanks the spirit for its assistance.

The Spiritual and Emotional Properties

Call on the spirit of the plant to help bring good fortune and luck. It brings warmth and love to one's heart. It helps to clear one's mind. It alleviates fear and anxiety and promotes a deep sense of faith and trust in oneself and one's purpose. Poke brings calmness and helps to heal one's spirit when it is broken. Call on this plant spirit to soothe your baby when it cries incessantly. Poke assists in the alignment of a person to their soul's intention. It is used for strength, especially when one is making leaps and bounds in their personal growth. It is good for protection when one is traveling. It is a very sacred plant. It is useful for the integration of one's emotional and mental faculties when there is much confusion. Use the plant spirit to help you call on your own spirit guides and helpers. It is useful in establishing healthy energetic boundaries between a parent and child. The plant spirit is used to honor the ancestors and elders who have come before us. It assists in the healing of the planetary consciousness.

The poke plant is used to induce trancelike or waking dream states of consciousness for purposes of healing. It also brings clarity to one's intuitive sense.

The Physical Healing Properties

Do not use when pregnant or nursing.

- Poke is useful for soothing throat irritation: mix drops of the essence with wheat germ oil and massage on the throat area.

- It is very helpful for hemorrhoids: make a mixture of drops of the essence and warmed olive oil and massage on the outside of the rectal area.

- For intestinal parasites, add 2–6 drops of the essence in warm water and drink sparingly. It is a very strong vibrational medicine. The tea can also be taken for intestinal and stomach cleansing.

- For muscle soreness, make a mixture of almond oil, drops of the essence, and lavender leaves and massage onto sore areas.

- For shallow breathing, massage a few drops of the essence and warmed olive oil onto the chest area.

- To heal the energies around strong influenza and tuberculosis, make a tea of 8–10 drops of the essence and hot water, adding a touch of honey and lemon.

- For mental illness and dissociative disorders, call on the spirit of the plant. Also call on the spirit to assist with Down's syndrome and intellectual disability. It will help to rebalance and recirculate the energy around the head.

- For anxiety and nervousness, take 4–6 drops of the essence three times a day until anxiety dissipates.

- For serious illness, call on the spirit of the plant to assist. The plant spirit essence helps with energetic and environmental sensitivities and helps to strengthen one's energy field.

CAUTION: Many parts of the poke plant are mildly poisonous and are not for consumption. It is to be handled by experienced practitioners and foragers only. When making the plant spirit essence, for your own safety, no part of the plant is to be harvested. Use the suggested prayer, meditate on the plant, and call on the plant spirit to imbue the essence with its healing properties.

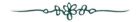

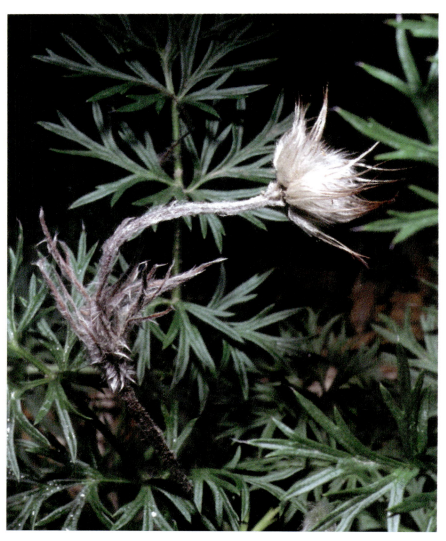

Pulsatilla

Plant Spirit Prayer

Oh, Holy of Holies, we beseech thee to embrace our prayers with the powers of Spirit, with the essence of God. We surrender before your discernment and ask for the grace of healing. We ask that our prayers be carried to heaven, upon the wings of the hummingbird, only to return with them answered in the will of the highest good.

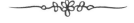

Pulsatilla
(*Anemone pulsatilla*)

My Experience with This Plant Spirit

In calling on the spirit of the plant, swooping down from amid the trees comes a darling little hummingbird. With vibrant markings of fuchsia, it flutters aimlessly around the beautiful purple petals that adorn the plant. It sticks its long beak into the yellow center of the flower and then hastily flies off into the sky, as though it were carrying something in its mouth. As it flies into the clouds, one can see that the hummingbird is carrying a prayer from a person that is securely placed within the loving embrace of pulsatilla's petals. As it nears the clouds, they begin to pull apart making a passageway for this little bird, with the sun shining ever so brightly. The sky becomes filled with brilliant rays of golden-yellow light and out of the ethers appear two magnificent hands—cupped and ready to receive the offerings that the hummingbird brings. The prayer gets gently placed into the hands of this holy one, where it is read with much compassion. If you listen closely enough, you will hear the voice belonging to these gifted hands. It is the voice of the miraculous St. Francis of Assisi. After answering the prayer, he holds it out for the hummingbird to grasp in its beak again to be brought back to the pulsatilla plant. The little hummingbird returns to the flower and places the prayer gently where he found it. Every time you see a hummingbird, remember your prayers are being answered.

The Spiritual and Emotional Properties

Call on the spirit of the plant to help you learn compassion and nonjudgment toward yourself and others. It helps you to learn to love yourself wholly and with complete acceptance of who you are. It helps when one is feeling melancholy and discontent. Use this plant when you are having much regret about your life; it helps you to understand the larger picture of why things unfolded the way they did. It helps to heal issues of abandonment of self and others. It helps assist one emotionally with the process of abortion and heals the energy field from this energetic trauma. The plant spirit also helps a person to take responsibility for one's actions toward others and to make amends with themselves around their actions. It gives one courage to heal. It fosters mutual respect in people. It nourishes and heals friendships. The pulsatilla plant is symbolic of the Christian celebration of Easter, of rebirth. It brings with it a new opening in one's life. It symbolizes the chance to begin anew. It is the plant of resurrection, of new and everlasting life. It is the promise of the Eternal Kingdom in the here and now and to come. It is a flower of hope and assists in healing deep despair.

The Physical Healing Properties

- Pulsatilla is good for headaches: take 2 drops of the essence every hour in water until the pain subsides.

- It helps heal the energy around chicken pox and shingles: place drops of the essence or fresh or dried flowers in a bath and soak.

- For dizziness, just smelling the flowers will help bring your energy back to the center.

- For low blood pressure, mix the essence with wheat germ oil and massage generously on the inside of your wrists, along the inside of feet, and over the breastbone.

- When your energy is low and it feels like the wind got knocked out of you, take 1–3 drops under your tongue.

- It helps to tonify the uterus and ovaries: massage a few drops of the essence along with warmed almond oil onto your pelvic area.

- It assists in bringing a normal menstrual flow when one is irregular (only at the time of menstruating). Make a compress using fresh or dried flowers and the leaves of pulsatilla and moisten them with a little olive oil. Massage the area first with warmed olive oil then place the leaves between folded layers of cotton cloth and lay it on the pelvic area for twenty to thirty minutes once a day. This is best done in the morning.

- Pulsatilla is excellent for anemia and low iron. Take 2 drops of the essence along with 2 drops of nettles essence to make an overall tonifying remedy.

- It is also good for tonifying the liver: make a mixture of wheat germ oil, castor oil, and few drops of the essence and massage over the liver. Adding heat for ten minutes or so will increase the benefits of this remedy.

- Call on the spirit of the plant to help balance your nervous system or take a drop of the essence under the tongue.

- It helps to alleviate some of the discomfort experienced with allergies to pollen. Upon waking, take 1–2 drops of the essence in water.

- It also helps to tonify the colon. Make an oil of fresh or dried flowers and olive oil and massage the warmed oil onto the lower back.

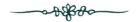

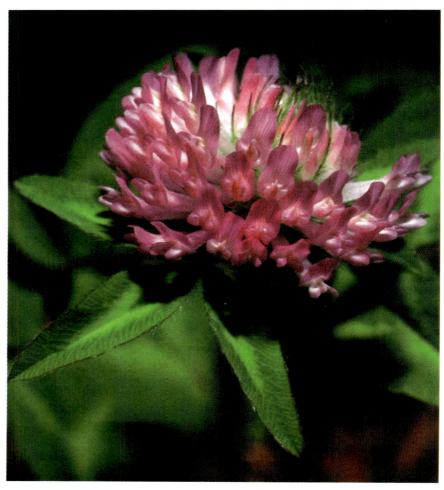

Red Clover

Plant Spirit Prayer

From the time of birth to the ending of life, may the cycle of Spirit never be broken. May the fire of God bless us and keep holy the path we walk.

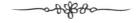

Red Clover
(*Trifolium pratense*)

My Experience with This Plant Spirit

In calling on the spirit of the plant, a strong and solemn male voice answers my prayer. This voice belongs to a spirit who incarnated on earth long ago. He works in alternate realities now in the spirit world, continuing with the work that he started many centuries ago. He shows me his hands, very strong and powerful, those of a healer. He used his hands to help heal many by laying them upon those who sought his help. He also counseled many in their troubles and made medicines from the plants to give to others. One evening, after a long day of hard work and assisting others, he sat at his washing bowl and submerged his hands into the water to cleanse himself of the energies of the day. He brought his hands cupped with some water to his face and quenched his tired skin. Upon finishing his ritual, he noticed in the bowl of water some markings that formed into a pattern. It resembled a flame, the fire of God. The healer started to weep at God's acknowledgment of his work and humbly thanked his Creator. He was so moved that he brought the water outside to nourish the many plants he works with, one of them specifically being red clover. He threw the remaining water over the red clover, and from that moment on, each leaf of the plant was marked with the symbol of the awesome fire of God. It is a very powerful healing plant.

The Spiritual and Emotional Properties

Call on the spirit of the plant to help heal pain and conflict between husband and wife. It also helps to heal your relationship with your mother and father. Red clover is used when one is feeling ashamed and unworthy. It is useful in healing anger in the heart space and to help one find forgiveness in the most challenging of situations. It gives one the courage to express themselves and share their innermost feelings.

Call on the spirit of the plant when there is great emotional distance between immediate family members. It helps to bring the family unit closer together and strengthens it. Red clover brings one courage when an apology is called for.

It is a plant of fortitude. It fosters determination, will, and persistence to keep going. It fosters honesty within a person and toward others. It helps when you are feeling angst and the loss of control over things in your life. It works to bring that sense of balance back.

It helps one to take responsibility for one's actions. Call on the plant spirit to bring you good luck when finding a job.

It will help to heal the energy when someone has been in a car accident.

Red clover is about honoring. It assists one in finding a sense of honor within themselves and toward others.

The Physical Healing Properties

- Red clover helps to heal the emotional energy around throat cancer: make an oil of fresh or dried flowers and St. John's wort oil and massage over the throat area. The essence may be used when flowers are not available.

- It is useful for sinus inflammation. Make an oil of wheat germ oil and fresh or dried flowers and massage the warmed oil over sinus passages.

- To improve circulation, throw some leaves and flowers into your hot bath, or massage over the body with warmed oil of fresh or dried flowers and olive oil.

- To tonify, purify, and cleanse the blood, take 3–6 drops of the essence in the morning under the tongue.

- It aids in healing the energy around lymphatic cancer: take 2–4 drops of the essence in warmed water upon waking per day and also place drops of the essence in your bath.

- To strengthen eyesight, take 1 drop of the essence under tongue upon waking.

- It also is a good remedy for combating the effects of the toxins from smoking: take 2–6 drops of the essence in water in the early afternoon.

- It helps to ease the pain of migraines: take 1 drop immediately under the tongue at the onset of pain.

- Red clover is excellent for healing the energy around the birth of a child through cesarean section. One can place the plant around you at night while sleeping, and also make an oil of fresh or dried flowers, leaves of lavender, and almond oil and massage onto the area of the uterus.

- For ectopic pregnancies, also use the same oil and massage onto the area of the uterus.

- The plant is sacred in that it nourishes the energy of the mother's breast milk while she is nursing. Just place plants of red clover around you during this time!

- It also nourishes the mother's system on a physical and energetic level after pregnancy. After the birth of the child and during the first year, take 1 drop of the essence in water when needed.

- It also helps reduce the discomfort of and aids in the energetic healing of breast polyps. Make a mixture of the essence and warmed olive oil and massage over the breasts.

- To ease lower back pain, massage a mixture of drops of the essence and almond oil onto the affected area.

- To assist the energetic healing of yeast infections, take 8–10 drops of the essence in water per day.

- For detoxifying the liver and kidneys, add a few drops of the essence to castor oil and make a castor oil pack to place over the kidneys and liver as needed.

- Red clover also strengthens the adrenals: make a mixture of warmed wheat germ oil, drops of the essence, and drops of rosemary essence and massage onto the adrenal area.

- It is also very useful in healing the energy surrounding general infections: take 10–20 drops of the essence in water per day.

- It is also helpful in removing toxicity from the body: take 3–5 drops of the essence in water per day.

- For worms and parasites, take 15 drops of the essence in water per day as needed upon retiring.

➤ It is very beneficial in healing the energy of all sexually transmitted diseases, such as gonorrhea, syphilis, and hepatitis. Take 15 drops of the essence per day under the tongue upon waking. Also massage a mixture of warmed St. John's wort oil and drops of the essence onto the pubic area.

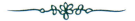

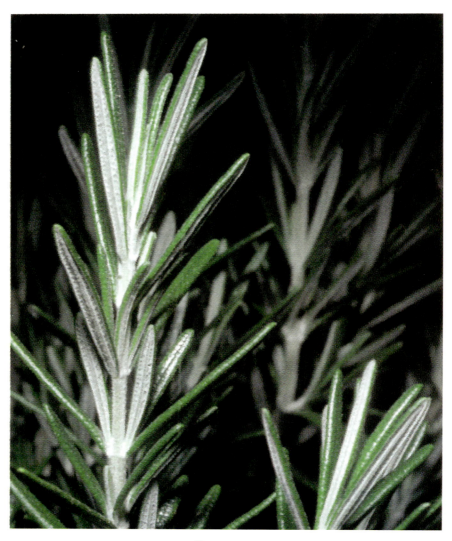

Rosemary

Plant Spirit Prayer

*Oh, Divine Mother, all loving, all knowing, and ever so present.
Fill our hearts with the grace of your love. Hold us in your tender arms.
Give to us divine mercy in our suffering. Be with us at the time of our
loneliness. Show us how to be compassionate with ourselves
and with humankind. Teach us the ways of God.*

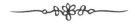

Rosemary
(*Rosemarinus officinalis*)

My Experience with This Plant Spirit

In calling on the spirit of the plant, one might hear the angelic voice of a little girl. She is soft and almost transparent in nature; and she nestles herself among the many flowers of her world. She is very connected with the energy of the Divine Mother, filled with so much unconditional love to give. She joyfully frolics along with no worries and not a care in the world, keeping to herself and tending to her flowers. She has always had a special relationship to them, especially the rosemary bush. Her love for them and for God transcends her everyday realities. As she comes close to the plant, she bends down, with her dress sweeping the dirt, and takes a piece, holding it tightly in her hand. She begins to talk with it, and as she does, behind her comes this magnificent ray of light, filled with golden-blue hues of vibrant warmth and radiance. The light embraces the little girl, and in it a form begins to emerge. The Divine Mother Mary, arms outstretched, envelops the child and the rosemary plant, imbuing both of them with her energy. The child's heart fills with a love so expansive that tears begin to fall from her cheeks. One of the tears falls upon the plant, giving it its healing properties.

The Spiritual and Emotional Properties

Call on the spirit of the plant to bring comfort when one is feeling alone and lonely. It brings quietness and stillness to one's life. It fosters understanding. It helps one to heal grudges held against another. It helps one to heal past resentments and bitterness toward another. Call on this plant to help you in forgiving your own past and making peace with yourself around it. It is essential in the forgiveness process on many levels. Rosemary will help you to let go and find that place inside yourself that gives you the courage to move on. It will aid you in reclaiming the present and opening to what the future has in store for you. It will help you to heal old wounds and to also forgive your parents. The Spirit of the plant is very connected to the Divine Mother energy. It brings such holiness into one's life and situations. It opens doorways into the higher self. It protects the home from intruders and is a wonderful protection against dark and negative energies. It assists you in staying present. It also assists in helping you create a vision for your future. To anoint oneself with rosemary is to be truly blessed by God.

The Physical Healing Properties

- Rosemary assists in shifting the energies associated with shallow breathing and congestion in the lungs due to smoking. Infuse the fresh or dried herb in almond oil and then massage onto the chest area. Also take a homeopathic dosage of 2–6 drops of the essence per day.

- For headaches, take 6 drops of the essence in water at the onset of the pain. For sinus trouble, make an oil of dried or fresh herbs and olive oil, and massage into affected area.

- It is very useful for stimulating the circulatory system: take 1 drop of the essence daily under the tongue in late morning to early afternoon.

- Drinking an infusion of the leaves is beneficial in lowering cholesterol.

- It is a very good remedy for detoxifying the liver. This can be done by drinking an infusion of the leaves as well.

- It helps to alleviate stomach acid. When stomach acid begins to be disruptive, massage a mixture of warmed olive oil and drops of the essence onto the gastrointestinal area.

- Rosemary also strengthens the immune system: take a homeopathic dosage of 1–3 drops of the essence when your system feels weakened. Also drinking a tea made from the infusion of the leaves will help.

- It is also beneficial for arthritis pain: make an oil with almond oil and fresh leaves and massage onto affected areas.

- To regulate blood sugar and nourish the spleen energy, massage a mixture of fresh or dried herb or drops of the essence with warmed wheat germ oil over the spleen and pancreas.

- For sore throats, make a mixture of the essence with olive oil and St. John's wort oil and massage over throat area.

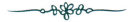

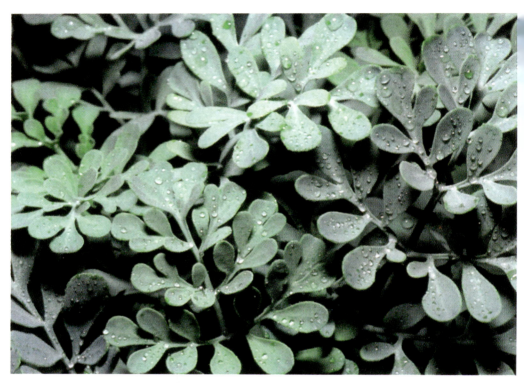

Rue

Plant Spirit Prayer

Almighty Spirit, bring us everlasting life as we embark on our journeys.
Heal us from the ills of self and protect our souls from harm.
We ask this in accordance with divine righteousness.

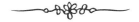

Rue
(*Ruta graveolens*)

My Experience with This Plant Spirit

In calling on the spirit of the plant, lightning and thunder roll across the sky. No apparition appears, yet an intense voice bursts forth from the loud roars of the heavens. This is the spirit of rue. He will never make himself shown to humans, only to that of the rue plant. The rue are like his children, for he nurtures them and grows them with much care. Every time a request for healing is made, the spirit sends heavy rains with brilliant showers of lightning bolts and bursts of thunder to each rue plant. The leaves, at the excitement of the forthcoming energies, raise themselves and their tips become gently graced with the light of this fiery and powerful essence.

The Spiritual and Emotional Properties

Call on the spirit of the plant to help with mental hysteria. It is useful when one is feeling disembodied. Rue is excellent in warding off evil spirits and negative energies, and it is used to draw out spirits that have inhabited a person's body. It assists one in crossing over into other dimensions. This is a very powerful plant and should be used with care!

Rue also facilitates healing and medicine dreams and altered states of consciousness.

It protects babies and fetuses inside the womb from harm. It protects those going on long journeys.

It is used when one is performing last rites on a dying person in any tradition to help protect their soul as it crosses over. Many spirits of the light are drawn to rue in reverence. It protects the etheric realm. It strengthens the etheric field in one's energy body.

The Physical Healing Properties

Do not use when pregnant or nursing.

- Rue is a good blood cleanser and improves circulation: take 4 drops of the essence in water upon waking.

- It helps heal the energy associated with rheumatoid arthritis and other joint and muscular pain. Make an oil of the leaves of rue steeped in olive oil and massage the warmed oil over painful areas of the body.

- It cleanses the arteries and improves blood and oxygen flow to the heart: take a drop of the essence in water upon waking. You can also massage the area of the heart with warmed St. John's wort oil, then take the fresh leaves and place on top of the heart area for ten to fifteen minutes.

- It helps alleviate nausea and also brings alkalinity to the stomach and digestive tract: make a compress of the fresh leaves moistened with a little warm water. Place the leaves between folded layers of cotton cloth and leave on the stomach for twenty-to-thirty-minute intervals.

- It is excellent for energetically maintaining homeostasis in the body and balancing the endocrine system: take 2 drops of the essence under the tongue as needed.

- It assists in healing the energy of Lyme disease. Place plants of rue around you or place a few drops of the essence in water and sip slowly on a daily basis.

- It draws toxins out of the liver, gallbladder, and kidneys. Massage the area first with a little warmed avocado oil then take the fresh leaves and place on top of intended areas.

- It balances the uterine energy and improves circulation in the uterus. Make an oil of the fresh leaves and almond oil and massage the warmed oil onto the pelvis.

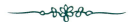

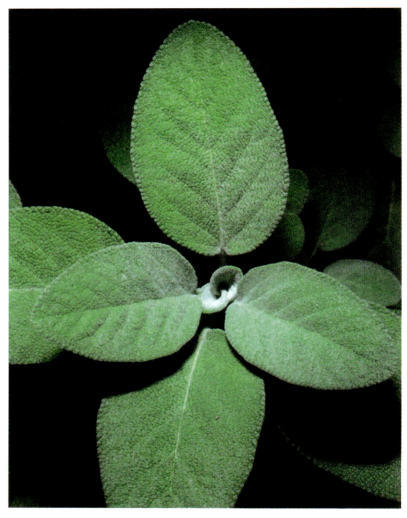

Sage

Plant Spirit Prayer

Grandmother, we open our arms to take in your wisdom. Let us not be foolish in our ways. Heal us from impatience and ignorance. Help us to walk the path of righteousness with Spirit. Guide us and help us to guide those who come after us.

We pray to you, oh grandmother, that we may be made humble to pass on your wisdom.

Sage
(*Salvia officinalis*)

My Experience with This Plant Spirit

In calling on the spirit of the plant, I heard the crackling voice of an elderly woman. She is a storyteller—a wise woman, gifted with tales passed down from one generation to the next. She is sitting at a potting wheel, one of her hobbies since a child. She is creating something, an object of beauty that will eventually be given to someone special. Surrounding her are children. They come from all over to hear her stories. She shares with the children about the importance of listening to their elders. She talks about how pride, envy, hatred, and jealousy can cause us to lose our spirits. She communicates the importance of loving one another and sharing what Spirit gave us. Most importantly, she reminds all of us, "Do unto others as we would like to have done unto us." She takes out the sage plant that she has had since she was a young one and passes it around to all the children to touch. She tells them that it was that very sage plant who taught her everything she knew, that passed down to her all of her most prized stories. She says each sage plant has a story to tell and if you listen closely, you will hear it. Ever since she passed on, her spirit stays close to the sage wherever it grows and helps others to hear its stories.

The Spiritual and Emotional Properties

Call on the spirit of the plant when you are holding anger or rage toward another. It will help you to heal it. It helps to heal hatred in a person. It helps to clear negative thoughts a person might be having by bringing the focus back to oneself. When one is seeking vengeance on another, call on the plant spirit to help you remember your spiritual self. It assists in clearing evil and darkness in persons, circumstances, and situations. It helps to bring insight and light to one's shadow side. It heals scorn and bitterness. It helps to ease the suffering that comes from feeling envy and jealousy, especially in personal relationships. It helps to heal strife and conflict between children. Call on the plant spirit to heal negative emotions between family members. It works to bring light to ego, self-righteousness, and pride.

It is one of the most powerful and sacred protectors against harm and evil spirits. It assists you in staying on your path and walking in the right direction. Sage represents karmic law, "what goes around, comes around" . . . this is one of sage's favorite stories to share with all of us.

The Physical Healing Properties

Do not use when pregnant.

- Sage is wonderful for quenching a thirst on a hot summer's day. Make an infusion of the leaves, add lemon and wildflower honey, cool it and enjoy.

- For colds and stuffy noses, take a dosage of 1–2 drops of the essence every hour until the symptoms clear.

- For coughs, take 3 drops of the essence every hour until the cough subsides. For swollen glands in the throat, make an oil with fresh or dried herbs and olive oil. Massage the warmed oil into the throat area.

- It is useful for lung congestion: take the essence and add it to warmed wheat germ oil and massage on the lungs.

- To strengthen the adrenals and kidneys, make a mixture of the essence, almond and wheat germ oils, and massage into kidney and adrenal areas.

- For increased overall muscular strength and muscle tone, massage a mixture of olive oil and dried or fresh herb into the muscles.

- To improve circulation within the digestive tract, make a compress with warmed olive oil and fresh or dried herb (fresh preferred here), and lay it on the stomach for twenty to thirty minutes. To make a compress, place the moistened herb between layers of folded cotton cloth. Do this late in the morning to early evening, leaving enough time between meals.

- Sage also helps to ease the discomfort of menstrual cramping and helps to regulate the menstrual cycle when it is irregular. For discomfort, take 2 drops of the essence in water upon waking. Do this during your cycle once a day until the cramping subsides. If your cycle is irregular, take 2 drops of the essence and mix it with almond oil and massage onto the pelvis.

- Sage also helps to heal the energy around varicose veins in the legs. Infuse almond oil with fresh leaves of sage and rosemary, leave it overnight when the moon is full, and massage it onto the legs for ten days. One also needs to pray to the plant spirit for help with this.

- When you need to feel more grounded, call on the plant spirit to assist with this. Taking 1 drop of the essence under the tongue when one feels ungrounded and placing a few drops of the essence 2 inches below the belly button will also help.

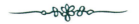

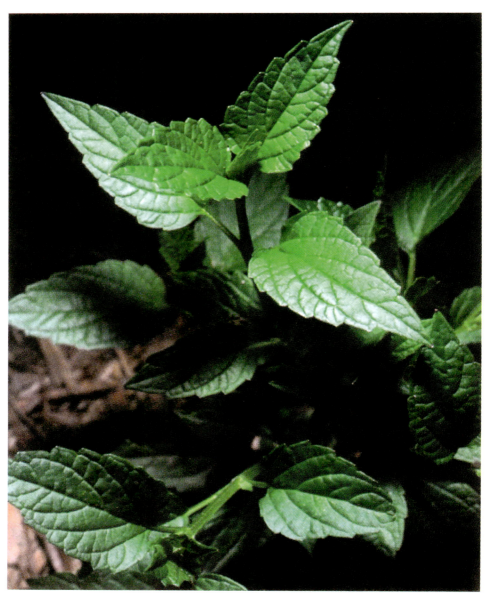

Skullcap

Plant Spirit Prayer

Rod of light, cast down upon us your invincible power of God.
Through the Holy Spirit, manifest truth of all things hidden and unseen.

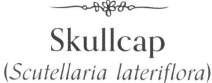

Skullcap
(*Scutellaria lateriflora*)

My Experience with This Plant Spirit

In calling on the spirit of the plant, a male spirit appears to me. He completed life on earth many years ago and before his passing, he left many things incomplete. From the moment he crossed over into the spirit world, he made a vow to assist others to uncover the truth in their lives and to bring light and completion to their experiences. He stands at the threshold of the clouds, a man of great stature. He holds in his hand a staff of invincible power. He will only help when he is called upon, acknowledging each person's free will to live their lives as they choose. He is a determined spirit though, and once his assistance is requested, he will raise his staff against the clouds and summon the winds to pull them apart. He then calls upon the skullcap plant to help in his endeavors. The plant willingly submits its presence, and the spirit takes his staff and directs the winds of power to touch the plant, thereby imbuing it with its healing abilities.

The Spiritual and Emotional Properties

Call on the spirit of the plant to help open the throat chakra. It gives one the courage to speak. It helps to heal the energetic trauma around deafness. For those whose expression was stifled in their younger years, call on skullcap to help you have a voice. It helps to heal insecurity and shyness. It helps to heal the energies around mental and physical disabilities. It works in the etheric field by healing the template that holds the structure upon which things manifest in the body. It heals the energetic trauma of cerebral palsy. It works to energetically balance brain function. Call on the spirit of skullcap when one is totally disconnected from Spirit by way of their intellect. It helps to unlock and unveil secrets that are destructive to one's spirit. It brings light and truth to secrets that have been withheld for a long time. It brings things to completion. It brings to light the unknown or hidden aspects of one's life in a safe and gentle way. It heals the energetic challenges around relationships between a brother and sister.

The Physical Healing Properties

- Skullcap is excellent for healing the energies around hay fever and allergies: take 4–6 drops of the essence in water a few times daily as needed.

- For pressure headaches, make a compress of the leaves of skullcap and place on top of the forehead for twenty-minute intervals. Do this by moistening the leaves with warm water and placing them between layers of folded cotton cloth.

- For phlegm in the throat and lungs, take a few drops of the essence in water as needed. Also, make a mixture of the essence in warmed almond oil and massage onto the chest and throat area. This remedy is also good when there is difficulty breathing that is associated with allergies.

- Skullcap acts as a natural sedative: place plants around you when you rest or take a drop of the essence under your tongue.

- For general irritability, take 2 drops of the essence in warmed water and sip slowly.

- For irritability associated with premenstrual syndrome, massage a generous amount of warmed olive oil mixed with drops of the essence onto the pelvis.

- It helps to heal the energy around tonsillitis: mix drops of the essence with St. John's wort oil and massage onto the throat area.

- For uterine cramping and as a natural relaxant for the uterine muscles, place plants of skullcap around you. Also, massage an infusion of the leaves of skullcap with almond and avocado oils onto the pelvis.

- It relieves vaginal burning and itching associated with viral infections: make a compress of the leaves of skullcap and place on top of pubic area for fifteen to twenty minutes. Do this by moistening the leaves with a little warmed olive oil and place it between layers of folded cotton cloth.

- It assists in alleviating the itching and toxins that come with insect bites: make a paste using a little bentonite clay, a touch of water, and drops of the essence and place on the affected areas. **Do not use on open sores.**

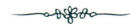

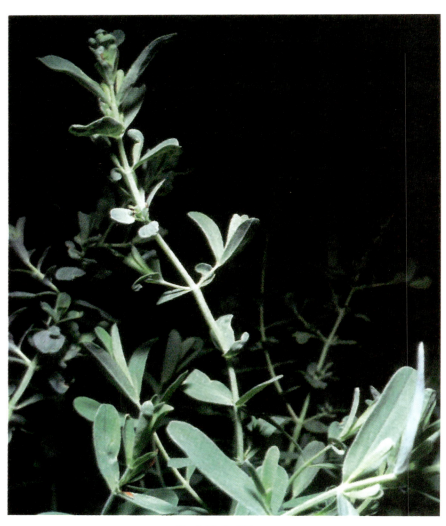

St. John's Wort

Plant Spirit Prayer

Divine Truth, shed for us the healing waters through your many tears. Shed for us the breath of life through your blood. Deliver us into the grace of eternal life. Grant us peace within.

St. John's Wort
(*Hypericum perforatum*)

My Experience with This Plant Spirit

In calling on the spirit of the plant, a miraculous vision comes into my sight of a beautiful garden filled with the flowering plants of St. John's wort. Their golden healing energy emanates to all the living creatures around it. The energy is so beautiful that many deer become drawn to sitting by it and sharing in its grace. This plant is sacred in that it is connected to St. John the Baptist and Jesus Christ. Whenever a prayer is requested of the saint, one can find him hovering over St. John's wort. With arms outstretched and serious intention in his eyes, he answers the many prayers that come. Blood sheds from his wrists into his hands and gently falls upon the leaves of St. John's wort. The plant becomes enveloped in this glowing and radiant red light. In its surrendering for a higher good, it begins to shed tears and also drops of red blood from its flowers and leaves. The blood is symbolic of the blood that Christ shed for humanity. It willingly gives itself over to Spirit to help heal many on a higher level of consciousness. As this unfoldment is taking place, the many creatures of the land come and surround the holy saint and the plant and sit among the healing energy that is gracefully emanating from it.

The Spiritual and Emotional Properties

The St. John's wort plant represents the bodhisattva, the realized creature that chooses to put off the kingdom of God to help others find their way home. It is excellent for healing depression. Call on the spirit of the plant when you are healing from the loss of a child. It helps to heal when one experiences any great loss in their lives. It heals the split in the heart space from overwhelming grief. It helps one to feel assured and more secure in one's life. It fosters self-confidence and self-esteem. It helps to create miracles in life by increasing faith. It helps turn around events in one's life and to become more positive when least expected. It brings many good blessings, light, and miraculous spiritual energy. It creates gentleness in animals. It enhances our connection with the Divine. It helps one to see clearly the path ahead and brings awareness. It is an excellent protection against evil spirits.

The Physical Healing Properties

- St. John's wort is excellent for healing the energy around spinal cord injuries, paralysis, and any other traumatic shock to the nervous system. Make an oil using the flowers of St. John's wort and add it to equal amounts of almond, olive, and grape-seed oils. Massage it onto the spine after bathing and before retiring.

- For healing the energy around blocked arteries, make an oil with the flowers and leaves, and equal amounts of grape-seed and borage oils, and massage onto the chest area.

- For headaches from poor nutrition, place 1 drop of essence under the tongue at the onset of discomfort. It would also be wise to examine your nutritional habits to prevent headaches in the future.

- For congestion and mucous in the throat, lungs, and gallbladder, make a tea using drops of the essence along with a touch of red clover essence.

- Massaging warmed olive oil mixed with the essence onto the lung area is also good for congestion.

- For congestion in the head and ear canals, drink the tea made with flowers of St. John's wort and also mullein leaves.

- It gently tonifies the immune system: take 2 drops of essence in water upon waking.

- To tonify the eyesight, make a compress of fresh or dried leaves and flowers moistened with water. Place between folded layers of cotton cloth and leave on the eyes for twenty-minute intervals.

- Placing the plant around you will induce sleep and bring calmness. To help ease anxiety, place a few drops of the essence under the tongue.

- It works to energetically balance an overactive thyroid: take 5 drops of the essence in water upon retiring.

- It helps to heal the energy of a prolapsed uterus. Lovingly massage warmed almond oil with drops of the essence onto your abdomen and pelvis.

- Massaging warmed wheat germ oil with a few drops of the essence will help to heal the pain of sciatica and also help energetically to manipulate a locked sacrum.

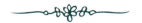

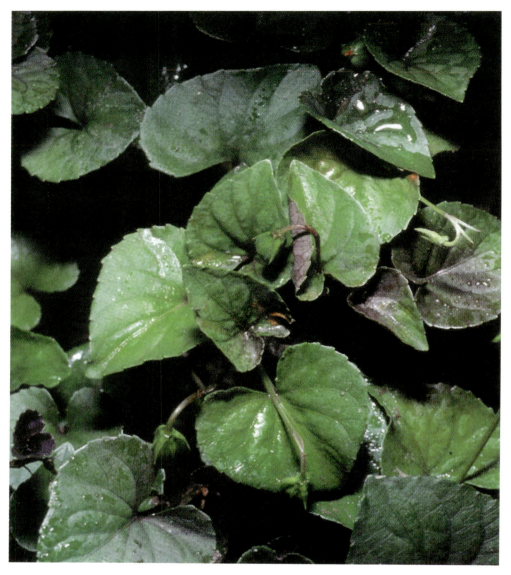

Violet

Plant Spirit Prayer

Oh Great Spirit, rest unto us your arms of nurturance and deliverance. In thy holy veil, grant us peace and harmony. Send forth your light to all those who seek your assistance and open us to the doors of heaven.

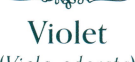

Violet
(*Viola odorata*)

My Experience with This Plant Spirit

In calling the spirit of the plant, a female essence appears to me. She is a luminescent one, bearing somewhat androgynous features. Ensconced in a flowing white robe, her hair drops down her back and nestles against her face. She is surrounded by beams of violet-blue light that cradle her every shadow. In her hand, she holds a beautiful white dove. This sacred bird carries in its beak a sprig of violet, as it lays wrapped in the essence of this spirit. Upon invoking the magic and healing of this plant, she sends the dove off to bring light and peace of heart to all those in need. The dove lays the sprig of violet in the spirits of all those who call to her for help. She is the plant spirit of harmony.

The Spiritual and Emotional Properties

Call on the spirit of the plant to help bring harmony when there is disharmony within a person's being. It also brings gentleness and the energy of simplicity when life becomes overwhelming. Violet creates joy and glee in one's life. It is soothing and calming when one has too many thoughts. It brings about a feeling of wholeness and centeredness. Violet is sacred in that it fosters compatibility, cooperation, and peace among people. It manifests light and brings a higher vibration to all those who call on this plant spirit for help. It heals emotional challenges and gently brings forth unconscious memories embedded from emotional trauma.

Violet has a very feminine nurturing energy and fosters self-assurance in a person. It increases one's intuition. Honoring this plant spirit will assist you in finding inner peace and peace within your relationships with others.

The Physical Healing Properties

- Violet is helpful in healing cramping associated with menstruation. Use the essence in a dosage of 2 drops in water every hour until the pain subsides. Combine the essence with St. John's wort oil and massage it gently into the pelvic area.

- For scratchy, watery eyes from allergens in the air, make a compress of the flowers and leaves and lay it on the eyes for ten-minute intervals. Do this by moistening the leaves with a little warmed water and placing them between layers of folded cotton cloth.

- To ease the soreness of foot calluses, mix 10 drops of the essence with equal amounts of warmed wheat germ oil, olive oil, and avocado oil.

- For drawing out the infection of boils on the skin, bathe with the leaves or add 30 drops of essence to bathwater while making a conscious connection to the plant spirit for help.

- For swollen glands in the throat area, massage the essence mixed with St. John's wort oil onto the affected area.

- For swollen lymph and pelvic glands, massage a mixture of almond oil and drops of the essence onto the affected areas.

- When there is acute inflammation as a result of chronic illness flare-up, take a dosage of 2 drops of the essence every hour in water.

- For jaw pain associated with dental work, lay a heavy compress on the inflamed area for an hour. Mix 3 tablespoons of dried herb with 1 clove of crushed garlic and 2 tablespoons of olive oil. Use a mortar and pestle and make a loose paste. Lay the mixture between folded layers of cotton cloth.

- To induce a restful sleep, surround yourself with fresh or dried flowers. To help with fatigue, take 12 drops of the essence per day between the hours of 11:00 a.m. and 1:00 p.m.

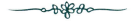

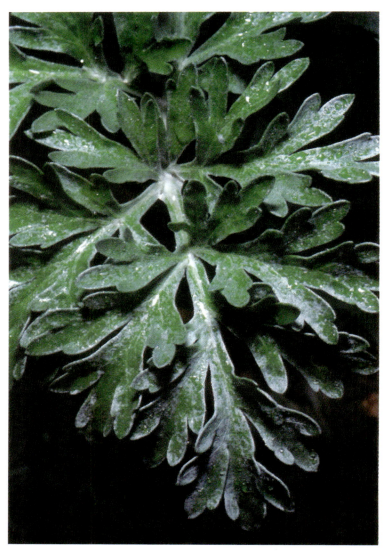

Wormwood

Plant Spirit Prayer

Oh Divine Providence, bring forth your spirit and help us to heal the many wounds of our hearts. We seek your refuge in our lives. Bring us back to our wombs, to the place where we are one with God to breathe in the fire of our souls.

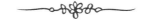

Wormwood
(*Artemisia absinthium*)

My Experience with This Plant Spirit

In calling on the spirit of the plant, a young maiden appears to me. Her face a gentle glow and hidden by her long, dark hair, she sits upon a rock with her hands laid gracefully by her sides. Her feet are enmeshed with the ground underneath her. She was born of the earth, a spirit of the lakes and rocks. She is bent over the side of a lake weeping sullenly for the loss of her lover and soul mate. She longs for him, searching and waiting for an eternity for his return. As her eyes gaze downward, she sees this silvery luminescent plant near her feet growing between the rocks. She reaches for it and cradles the plant in her arms like a child. Her many tears fall upon the leaves of this plant and activate its spirit. Its magic, essence, and spiritual healing properties spring forth with life. The young maiden uses the plant spirit essence to soothe her soul and call back her soul mate.

The Spiritual and Emotional Properties

Call on the spirit of the plant when you are feeling disconnected from your heart and inner guidance. By holding the plant up to one's heart chakra, the energy field surrounding the leaves permeates the heart membrane, increasing energy flow between the organ itself and the subtle energy layers that surround it.

It assists the healing process when one is devastated from the loss of a loved one. The loss of a soul mate or life partner can bring much agony;

calling on the spirit of wormwood can help one find peace within. It is excellent in healing grief. When one is having trouble in a relationship, call on the spirit of the plant to assist with healing at the heart level. Wormwood is essential in healing the loss of a child and also miscarriages. When one loses a child, cradling the plant itself in one's arms helps to nourish and heal the grief. When there is a miscarriage, many times the spirit of the unborn baby is still with the mother. The mother's healing is around letting go of the spirit and giving the child permission to cross over to the spirit world to continue on its journey. The spirit of the plant will assist the unborn baby to find its way to the light. Call on wormwood to soothe irritability in children whatever the cause. It brings about playfulness and jovialness.

The plant spirit also aids in crossing over souls who have already separated from their physical bodies due to death but are not ready to fully transition and are confused about where they are. By placing the plant and a white candle near the deceased and through intention, the souls will feel more at peace with transitioning to their next place of being. Wormwood is excellent in warding off evil spirits and for protection. It is blessed by the spirit world and held in high regard for this purpose. On an energetic level, the spirit of wormwood helps to align the crown chakra, the Divine light of God, and clears the heart at the soul center, drawing the energy downward and healing the physical body.

The Physical Healing Properties

Do not use when pregnant or nursing.

- Wormwood is excellent in tonifying and energetically clearing the mucous in glands that become swollen. It also aids in energetically clearing the lymphatic system: take 4 drops of the essence in water upon waking.

- It eases the pain and inflammation of arthritis, rheumatic pain, and traumatic injury to the joints. It also helps to relieve back pain and tenderness from sciatica: make a mixture of the essence, warmed olive oil, and fresh parsley and massage onto affected areas.

🌿 To heal the energy around astigmatism and vision problems, lay a compress over the closed eyes for no longer than fifteen minutes. Do this by taking the leaves and moistening them with a little warmed water. Then place them between folded layers of cotton cloth. This is best done in the evening before you retire.

🌿 For a heart murmur, sleep with the plant over your heart at night and the glorious maiden will help it to heal.

🌿 For a vaginal yeast infection, take fresh chopped wormwood leaves and add a minuscule amount of warmed water and apply it directly over the pubic bone in the hour between 11:00 a.m. and noon. Leave it for a half hour to an hour depending upon the severity of the infection.

🌿 For a bladder infection, do the same as above and place the leaves right above the pubic bone for an hour between 2:00 and 3:00 in the afternoon. (Note: if you work outside the home, do these whenever you can.)

🌿 For parasites in the digestive tract, the essence helps to strengthen the boundary between the physical tissue and the parasites, assisting them in leaving the body. Place 4 drops of the essence in water and take upon retiring.

🌿 A few drops of the essence help to bring about mental clarity when brain fog is present.

🌿 It nourishes the blood, spleen, and heart energy and is good for grounding the etheric body into the earth. Place a drop of the essence under your tongue as needed.

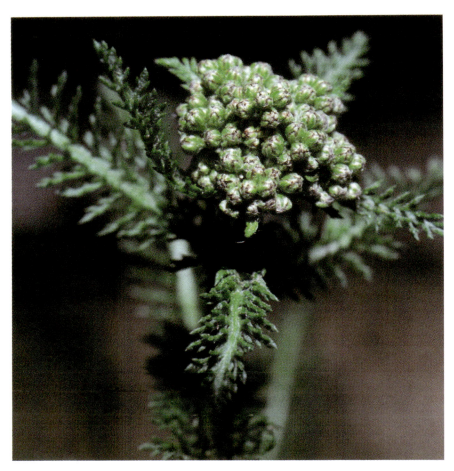

Yarrow

Plant Spirit Prayer

Oh glorious melody, upon your strings, enchant us with divine harmony.
And unto us, heal the fruits of our many labors.

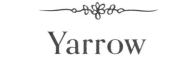

Yarrow
(*Achillea millefolium*)

My Experience with This Plant Spirit

In calling on the spirit of the plant, an innocent and gentle female spirit comes floating toward me. She is very ethereal, wearing a covering of white satin pressed against her long golden hair. She carries with her a harp, very surreal and enchanting. Upon hearing the healing cries of the yarrow plant, she gracefully sets herself down upon the earth in the midst of a lush green garden. Surrounding her are beautiful plants of yarrow that immediately become hypnotized by her majestic presence. They share their many requests for medicinal and spiritual healing from the outside world. The spirit begins to play a song, a melody for each request to be granted. As the music plays, the yarrow plants bend their stems toward this ethereal being, and the vibration of the music harmonizes the yarrow's incredible healing abilities.

The Spiritual and Emotional Properties

Call on the spirit of the plant when one is feeling discouraged. It is the plant of support and will foster that quality within one. When one is feeling alone in a situation or needing to stand up for oneself, family, or friends, call on yarrow to assist you. It will help you to get along with your neighbors. Yarrow will guide you in your life and will also guide you on the path of righteousness. Yarrow fosters emotional and mental support in a person. When one needs to explain oneself in a difficult situation, call on yarrow to bring you courage, comfort, and ease. Yarrow helps one to confront the truth in oneself and with others and to take responsibility for one's feelings. Yarrow can help when one is feeling disillusioned with one's life and work. Call on this plant spirit when you are feeling incompetent, devalued, and unable to live up to others' expectations, for yarrow can foster an amazing sense of self-worth. It also helps to heal the emotional and spiritual energies around learning disabilities and Alzheimer's disease.

The Physical Healing Properties

- Yarrow nourishes the energy of the spleen and pancreas: take 3 drops of the plant spirit essence under the tongue upon waking.

- It is excellent for cleansing mercury toxicity and poisoning of the blood from chemical toxicity: take 4 drops of the essence in water three times a day until condition improves. It is also a good lymphatic cleanser: take 2 drops in water when the need arises. It helps to cleanse environmental toxins both internally and in one's energy field. There are a few ways to assist with this. One can make a spray mist using the essence and moisten yourself with it. One can also take 5–10 drops of the essence in water when feeling overwhelmed from environmental sensitivities.

- Yarrow is excellent in healing the energy around many different infections. For infections and poisons in the uterus and cervix, make an oil with leaves of yarrow in almond oil and massage onto pelvis.

- For healing the energy around lung infections, pneumonia, and bronchitis, take 5–7 drops of the essence in water each hour until condition improves. Also massage an oil made from the leaves of yarrow, parsley, and olive oil onto chest area.

- It also is good for clearing infections of the ear canals: make a mixture of warmed olive oil, drops of yarrow essence, and red clover essence, and massage around the ears.

- To assist the healing of pink eye, make a compress using fresh leaves of yarrow moistened with a little warmed water. Place the plant material between folded layers of cotton cloth and place on closed eyes for twenty-minute intervals.

- It is also good for throat infections such as tonsillitis. Make an oil with the leaves and a few drops of essence with a combination of warm castor oil and olive oil and massage onto the throat area.

- It is useful in cleansing liver and gallbladder toxicity. Add a few drops of the essence to warm castor oil and massage onto these areas, or use with a castor oil pack.

- It helps to heal poisonous bites from insects: make a paste of the fresh cut leaves of yarrow with a small amount of bentonite clay and put on insect bites. **Do *not* use this with open sores**.

- It helps to heal the energy around fibroids and uterine cysts and cysts in the breast tissue. Make an oil with almond oil and leaves of yarrow and red clover and massage onto affected areas.

- Adding a drop of the essence to your water will nourish the blood.

- 🌿 It also helps to heal the pain of fibromyalgia. Add drops of the essence to your bathwater and also massage an oil made from yarrow leaves and warmed almond oil onto your body after bathing.

- 🌿 It is a good tonifier of the kidneys and adrenals. Place a few drops of the essence on your hands and just directly touch the part of your back where kidneys and adrenals sit.

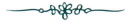

Guide to the Power of Plants

Physical Properties

Adrenals–lavender, lemon balm, licorice, red clover, sage, yarrow

Allergies–lemon balm, pulsatilla, skullcap

Anemia–nettles, pulsatilla

Anxiety–astragalus, poke, St. John's wort

Arteries–dandelion, rue, St. John's wort

Arthritis–blessed thistle, mullein, nettles, rosemary, rue, wormwood

Autoimmune Disease–motherwort

Babies–lamb's ear

Bladder–black cohosh, blessed thistle, lavender, licorice, mugwort, wormwood

Blood–blessed thistle, clematis, nettles, red clover, rue, wormwood, yarrow

Blood Pressure–angelica, blessed thistle, dandelion, pulsatilla

Blood Sugar–lilac, marshmallow, rosemary

Bones–chamomile

Brain Aneurysms–motherwort

Brain Function–blessed thistle, calendula, marshmallow, motherwort, skullcap, wormwood

Breast Cancer–black cohosh

Breast Polyps–red clover

Bruises, Cuts, Wounds–astragalus, mugwort

Burns–lavender

Cancers (Various)–black cohosh, lamb's ear, red clover

Cervical Cancer–black cohosh

Cervical Dysplasia–dandelion

Chicken Pox/Shingles–pulsatilla

Cholesterol–rosemary

Circulation–blessed thistle, dandelion, lilac, lemon balm, marshmallow, red clover, rosemary, rue, sage

Colds–sage

Colic–angelica

Colon–marshmallow, motherwort, nettles, pulsatilla, sage

Constipation–clematis, lemon balm

Convulsions–astragalus, chamomile, skullcap

Coughs–sage

Diaper Rash–chamomile, mullein

Diarrhea–chamomile, licorice

Digestive System–lavender, lemon balm, licorice, marshmallow, mugwort, nettles, sage

Dizziness–pulsatilla

Ears–feverfew, mugwort, St. John's wort, yarrow

Endocrine System–lamb's ear, rue

Energy–licorice, pulsatilla

Environmental Sensitivities/Toxicity–mullein, poke, yarrow

Eyes–blessed thistle, lamb's ear, lavender, mugwort, red clover, St. John's wort, violet, wormwood, yarrow

Fatigue–lemon balm

Feet–violet

Fertility–feverfew, astragalus

Fevers–angelica, feverfew

Fibroids/Cysts–black cohosh, red clover, yarrow

Fibromyalgia–yarrow

Fluid Retention–dandelion, mugwort

Fungus–clematis, lavender

Gallbladder–astragalus, blessed thistle, calendula, lilac, marshmallow, nettles, rue, St. John's wort, yarrow

Genital Herpes–clematis

Grounding–sage, wormwood

Hay Fever–skullcap

Headaches/Migraines–angelica, chamomile, dandelion, feverfew, pulsatilla, red clover, rosemary, skullcap, St. John's wort

Head Congestion–lemon balm, sage, St. John's wort

Heart–angelica, astragalus, black cohosh, blessed thistle, calendula, lamb's ear, motherwort. wormwood

Hemorrhoids–marshmallow, poke

Hernia–black cohosh

Hormones–astragalus, lilac

Immune System–astragalus, blessed thistle, motherwort, nettles, rosemary, St. John's wort, violet

Impotence–feverfew

Incontinence–mugwort

Indigestion–lavender, mugwort

Infections–red clover, yarrow

Influenza–chamomile, poke

Injuries–calendula

Insect Bites–skullcap, motherwort

Intestines–clematis, lemon balm, nettles

Jaw Pain–violet

Joints–calendula, mugwort, wormwood

Kidneys–blessed thistle, calendula, lavender, lemon balm, licorice, lilac, mugwort, mullein, red clover, rue, sage, yarrow

Learning Disabilities–feverfew

Liver–blessed thistle, feverfew, lavender, licorice, motherwort, nettles, pulsatilla, red clover, rosemary, rue, yarrow

Lungs (Breathing Ailments, Infections)–dandelion, feverfew, lemon balm, licorice, lilac, mullein, nettles, poke, rosemary, sage, skullcap, St. John's wort, yarrow

Lyme Disease–rue

Lymphatic Cancer–red clover

Lymphatic System–lavender, lilac, motherwort, nettles, violet, wormwood, yarrow

Menopause–lilac

Menstruation–angelica, black cohosh, blessed thistle, lavender, lilac, mugwort, nettles, pulsatilla, sage, skullcap, violet

Mental Illness–black cohosh, poke

Miscarriage—clematis

Morning Sickness—licorice, sage

Mucous—dandelion, lemon balm, mugwort, St. John's wort, wormwood

Multiple Sclerosis—mullein

Muscles—calendula, chamomile, motherwort, poke, sage

Nausea—chamomile, feverfew, rue

Nerve Pain—calendula, feverfew

Nervous System—angelica, astragalus, black cohosh, motherwort, pulsatilla, St. John's wort

Nosebleeds—black cohosh

Pancreas—lavender, lilac, marshmallow, motherwort, yarrow

Parasites—calendula, marshmallow, poke, red clover, wormwood

Poison Ivy/Oak—chamomile

Pregnancy/Birthing—red clover

Prickly Heat—mullein

Rape/Sexual Violence—lamb's ear

Reproductive System (Males)—angelica, lamb's ear

Rest/Sedation—motherwort, skullcap, St. John's wort, violet

Scar Tissue—motherwort

Sciatica–St. John's wort, wormwood

Seizures–clematis, lamb's ear

Sexual Energy–calendula

Sexually Transmitted Diseases–red clover

Sinus–dandelion, lavender, licorice, mugwort, nettles, red clover, rosemary

Skeletal-Muscular System–blessed thistle

Skin Rashes/Diseases–chamomile, clematis, marshmallow, mullein, violet

Smoking–lemon balm, rosemary

Spinal Column–motherwort, St. John's wort

Spleen–lavender, marshmallow, motherwort, rosemary, wormwood, yarrow

Stomach–astragalus, nettles, rosemary, rue

Strength–nettles

Stress–black cohosh, lemon balm, lavender

Swollen Glands–sage, violet, wormwood

Throat–astragalus, feverfew, lemon balm, poke, rosemary, sage, skullcap, St. John's wort, yarrow

Throat Cancer–red clover

Thymus–blessed thistle, calendula

Thyroid–lamb's ear, St. John's wort

Tonsillitis–skullcap

Toothache–chamomile

Tumors–motherwort

Ulcers–marshmallow, motherwort

Uterus–angelica, black cohosh, calendula, lemon balm, pulsatilla, rue, skullcap, St. John's wort, violet, yarrow

Vaginal Discomfort–skullcap

Varicose Veins–sage

Weakness–mullein

Worms–clematis, feverfew, red clover, wormwood

Yeast Infections/Candida–clematis, lavender, lilac, red clover, wormwood

Spiritual and Emotional Properties

Abandonment–calendula, motherwort, pulsatilla

Abortion–pulsatilla

Abundance/Finances–dandelion, feverfew, poke

Abuse–dandelion, lamb's ear, mugwort

Acceptance–dandelion, lamb's ear, pulsatilla

Addictions–chamomile

Adoption–black cohosh

Alcoholism–chamomile, mugwort

Alzheimer's Disease–yarrow

Ancestral Honoring–poke

Anger/Rage–chamomile, nettles, red clover, rosemary, sage

Animals–black cohosh, lilac, St. John's wort

Anxiety–marshmallow, poke

Authority–marshmallow

Balance–marshmallow

Boundaries–angelica, astragalus, calendula, poke

Celebration–blessed thistle

Ceremony–black cohosh

Child Labor–licorice

Child Loss–black cohosh, pulsatilla, St. John's wort, wormwood

Children/Babies–blessed thistle, calendula, lamb's ear, lemon balm, motherwort, mugwort, poke, rue, sage, wormwood

Codependency–blessed thistle

Comfort–astragalus, calendula, licorice, lilac, rosemary, yarrow

Communing with Spirit World/Higher Power–lavender, mugwort, mullein, poke, rue

Community–clematis

Compassion–blessed thistle, clematis, pulsatilla

Compatibility–violet

Completion–blessed thistle, skullcap

Compromise–feverfew

Concentration–blessed thistle

Conflict–mullein, red clover

Confusion–chamomile, marshmallow, poke

Courage–lemon balm, pulsatilla, red clover, skullcap

Creativity–feverfew

Cultural/World Consciousness–clematis, licorice, poke

Deafness (Trauma Surrounding It)–Skullcap

Desire–mugwort

Direction–motherwort

Disconnection from Self/Spirit–poke, skullcap, wormwood

Divine Mother–rosemary

Dreaming–poke, rue

Dying–mugwort, rue, wormwood

Elderly–blessed thistle

Emotional Stress–angelica, chamomile, marshmallow, mullein, violet

Empathy–nettles

Encouragement–mullein

Energy Field–angelica, lavender

Ethers–rue

Evil–angelica, black cohosh, feverfew, marshmallow, mugwort, rosemary, rue, sage, St. John's wort, wormwood

Expression–clematis, skullcap

Faith–mullein, poke

Fear–lemon balm, poke

Forgiveness–blessed thistle, lamb's ear, mullein, red clover, rosemary

Gentleness–violet

Grace–motherwort

Grief/Depression–chamomile, dandelion, feverfew, lavender, lemon balm, lilac, pulsatilla, red clover, rosemary, St. John's wort, wormwood

Grounding–astragalus, nettles, rosemary, rue

Grudges–rosemary

Guidance–yarrow

Happiness–lavender, lilac, violet

Harmony–violet

Hatred–sage

Heartache–lemon balm

Honor–feverfew, red clover

Hope–licorice, pulsatilla

Injustice–lemon balm

Inner Child–calendula

Innocence–calendula

Insecurity–feverfew, skullcap, St. John's wort

Intuition–lamb's ear, sage, violet

Irritability–blessed thistle, wormwood

Jealousy/Envy–clematis, nettles, sage

Joy–calendula, lavender

Judgment–clematis, pulsatilla

Karma–lavender, licorice, sage

Light–feverfew, skullcap, violet, yarrow

Loneliness–calendula, rosemary, yarrow

Loss–astragalus, lamb's ear, lavender

Love–clematis, lamb's ear, lavender, lilac, poke, pulsatilla

Luck–poke, red clover

Magic–mullein

Menopause–lilac

Mental Hysteria–rue

Miracles–St. John's wort

Miscarriage–wormwood

Motivation–marshmallow, mugwort

Negative Thoughts–nettles, sage

Nervousness–angelica

Offering–black cohosh

Peace–blessed thistle, lamb's ear

Physical and Mental Disabilities–skullcap

Planetary Healing–poke

Play–calendula

Power–marshmallow

Pride–chamomile

Protection–angelica, black cohosh, blessed thistle, chamomile, feverfew, lamb's ear, marshmallow, motherwort, mugwort, poke, rosemary, rue, sage, St. John's wort, wormwood

Psychic Protection–angelica

Rape/Sexual Violence–lamb's ear, mugwort

Recovery–blessed thistle

Regret–feverfew, marshmallow, pulsatilla

Relationships–astragalus, blessed thistle, calendula, dandelion, feverfew, lavender, lilac, mullein, nettles, pulsatilla, red clover, sage, skullcap, violet, wormwood

Resentment–rosemary

Respect–astragalus, pulsatilla

Responsibility–pulsatilla, red clover

Resurrection–pulsatilla

Reverence–astragalus, black cohosh

Romance–lilac

Safety–calendula, chamomile, mullein

Secrets–skullcap

Self-Esteem–clematis, St. John's wort

Selfishness–clematis, nettles

Sensuality/Sexuality–calendula, lamb's ear

Shame–red clover

Shyness–lamb's ear, skullcap

Societal Issues–clematis, lamb's ear, licorice, motherwort, mugwort

Soul Loss–astragalus

Spiritual Aspiration–lemon balm

Strength–angelica, dandelion, lemon balm, poke, red clover

Support–licorice, mullein, yarrow

Suppression–licorice

Surrendering–lamb's ear

Transition–lilac

Trauma–black cohosh, dandelion, lamb's ear, licorice, skullcap

Trust–poke

Truth–feverfew, skullcap, violet, yarrow

Unconscious Memories–violet

Understanding–dandelion, lamb's ear, pulsatilla, rosemary

Vengeance–sage

Violence–mugwort

Wars–licorice

Worry–mullein

Index

abandonment, 114
abortion, 140
abuse, 33, 75, 114
acceptance, 167
addictions, 151–52
adoption, 140
adrenal glands, 172–73, 177, 180, 218, 252
afterlife, 2
air element, 108
alcohol, 121
alcoholism, 151, 195
Alexis (cat), 81, 82, 91–96
allergies, 177, 196, 213, 234, 242
almond oil, 132, 141, 149, 157
alternate realities, 71
ancestors, 139
ancestral DNA, 3
anemia, 213
aneurysms, 192
angelica, *130*, 131–33
anger, 199, 229
angina, 132
animal spirits, 68–72

antibiotic, 132
anxiety, 137, 209
arteries, 160, 226, 238
arthritis, 145, 201, 205, 223, 226, 246
asthma, 42, 180, 200
astragalus, *134*, 135–37
Aversano, Laura
    beginning of spiritual path, 2–4
    client work, 105–6, 112–15
    connecting with Native American spirits, 59–69
    flower essences and, 87–89
    gathering plants, 82–87
    healing magic and, 10–17
    home garden of, 58–59
    karmic healing response, 25–30
    lost children and, 31–42
    medicine dream of, 76–78
    meeting John, 18–24
    miasm and, 14–15
    mother of, 4
    pesticides and, 87–92
    plant journeys of, 126–29

Index

shaman and, 5–9, 13–14, 21–24
writing of, 72–74, 84, 86

baths, 25, 36–38
beauty, 100
Becky (client), 42–47
beech, 72
bitterness, 203
black cohosh, 77–78, 93, 114–15, *138*, 139–41
Black Elk, 11, 88–89
bladder, 141, 145, 173, 181
blessed thistle, 93, *142*, 143–45
blood, 145, 157, 204, 217
blood cleanser, 226
blood pressure, 160, 212
blood sugar, 189, 223
bonds of light, 116–17
bone density, 152
boundaries, 44, 47, 114, 131, 136, 144
brain function, 144, 148, 188, 247
brandy, 121
breast cancer, 141
breast milk, 217
breast polyps, 218
broken hearts, 172
bronchitis, 42, 43, 184
bruises, 137
Buddha, 104, 109
burial rituals, 4
burns, 172
butterflies, 151

calendula, 82–84, *146*, 147–49
call, 6
calm, 151
cancer, 49–57, 169, 216, 217
candida, 184
canker sores, 156
Catholicism, 12, 44
Ceara (cat), 81, 82, 95
celebrations, 132
cemeteries, 18
cerebral palsy, 234
ceremony, 69
cervical cancer, 141
cervix, 149, 160
cesarean sections, 217
chamomile, *150*, 151–53
chemotherapy, 55
chest colds, 184
chest pain, 141
chicken pox, 212
children, 73–76, 78–79, 147–48
chills, 164
cholesterol, 222
circulation, 160, 177, 184, 188, 217, 231
clairaudience, 14
clairsentience, 14
clematis, 93, *154*, 155–57
codependency, 144
coffee grinds, 26–28
Coleridge, Samuel Taylor, 48
colic, 132
colon, 188, 205, 213
community, 155
compassion, 212
concentration camps, 33
conflict, 216, 230
confusion, 151
congestion, 165, 238–39
constipation, 156, 177
convulsions, 136, 152
coughs, 230

courage, 175
Crazy Horse, 11
Creator, 70
curses, 115, 131
cuts, 137
cysts, 141

dandelion, 85–87, *158*, 159–61
deer spirits, 61
demons, 113
depression, 151, 159, 238
devas, 6–7
diabetes, 161
diaper rash, 152, 200
diarrhea, 152
diet, 25
digestion, 181, 188, 196, 204
dishonesty, 155
dissociative disorders, 209
divination tools, 69
Divine, 98–106
Divine Chaplet, 20
Divine Mother, 37, 222
Divine Providence, 117–18, 128
divorce, 148
dizziness, 212
DNA, 3
droughts, 140
dryness, 196
duality, 131
dying, 152

ear infections, 164
ears, 196, 251
Earth, 103, 128
earth element, 108
ectopic pregnancies, 217

eczema, 201
elderly man (spirit), 135–36
elderly woman (spirit), 39–40
electrolytes, 136
elementals, plant, 6–8
elves, 6–7
emphysema, 200
emptiness, 16–17
endocrine system, 169, 226
energetic bonds of light, 116–17
energetic shields, 43
energy, 100–101
energy sensitivity, 112–13
entities, 114–15
environmental illness, 112–13
epileptic seizures, 157, 168
etheric body, 115–16
etheric mist, 15
Eve, Gospel of, 75
evil spirits, 139
evolution, personal, 116–17
expression, 155, 233–34
eyes and eyesight, 144, 168, 173, 196, 217, 239, 247, 251

fairies, 6–7, 61–62
faith, 116, 118, 207–8, 238
fatigue, 175, 177
feminine, 48–49, 135
fertility, 165
feverfew, 93, *162*, 163–65
fevers, 132, 164
fibroids, 141
fibromyalgia, 252
financial burdens, 164
fire element, 108
fires, 75, 78, 140

Flat Iron, 110
floods, 140
flower essences, 87–88
flowers, 98, 101–2
flu, 152, 209
fluid retention, 161, 196
flute music, 66
forgiveness, 199
fortitude, 216
four elements, 108
Francis of Assisi, St., 211
frustration, 132
fungus, 156

gallbladder, 25, 137, 144, 149, 184, 189, 205, 227, 251
gallstones, 137
gatherings, 132
genital herpes, 156
God, 4, 36, 47–48, 64, 98
Goddess, 98
gold coins, 159
good fortune, 207
Gospel of Eve, 75
grace, 99–100
gratitude, 110–11, 118
Great Mother, 77
Great Spirit, 69
Gregory of Nyssa, 102
grief, 159, 163, 184
Griffin, Susan, 70
grounding, 117, 231
guides, 69
Gurney, Dorothy Francis, 101

Hardin, Jesse Wolf, 129
harmony, 241

headaches, 132, 152, 160, 164, 212, 217, 222, 234, 238
head injuries, 136
healing, 100, 103, 116–19
healing crisis, 25–30
heart, 137, 145, 148, 175
heart attacks, 132, 168, 192
heart murmurs, 193
heat, 71, 75
hemorrhoids, 208
herpes, 156
high blood pressure, 132
higher power, 200
Higher Power, 16–17
Highest Will, 118
hip injuries, 149
hormones, 137
hot flashes, 185
Huainanzi, 103
human beings, 99–100
hummingbirds, 211
hypersensitivity, 131
hysteria, 140, 225

Ida (seer), 26–28
illness, 115–16
immune system, 137, 144, 223
impotence, 165
indigestion, 173, 196
infections, 218, 250–51
infertility, 140
inflammation, 180, 188, 242
influenza, 152, 209
initiations, 69
injustice, 175
insect bites, 235, 251
intention, 117–18

intestinal yeast, 156, 172, 184
intestines, 205
invocation prayer, 107–8
iron, low, 213
irritability, 132, 185, 234
itching, 71, 75

jaw pain, 243
jealousy, 155, 204
John (spirit), 18–24, 31, 38, 94, 95, 96
John the Baptist, St., 44
joint injuries, 149, 246
Joseph, St., 12
journey, preparing for, 107–11
joy, 100, 147

karma, 74, 112–13, 115
kidneys, 145, 148, 172–73, 177, 180, 185, 218, 227, 231, 252
knee injuries, 149

lamb's ear, 103–4, 167–69, *168*
lavender, *170*, 171–73
learning disabilities, 165
leaves, 101–2
lemon balm, 23–24, *174*, 175–77
leprechauns, 27
lethargy, 200
letting go, 116, 168
libido, 148
licorice, *178*, 179–81
light energy, 104
lilac, *182*, 183–85
liver, 25, 144, 172–73, 181, 205, 213, 218, 223, 227, 251
loneliness, 221
loss, 160

lost children, 11–13, 15, 31–42, 62, 94, 96
Lou Gehrig's disease, 192
love, 99–101, 121, 155
lower worlds, 136
luck, 207
lungs, 160, 165, 176, 200, 230
Lyme disease, 227
lymphatic system, 172, 204

Maria (mother), 43, 45–46
marshmallow, *186*, 187–89
masculine, 48–49, 135
massacre, 75–76
mass killings, 61, 75–76
Mayan prayer, 119
medicine men, 64–65
medicine women, 76–77
menopause, 185
menstruation, 132, 140, 145, 173, 185, 197, 204, 213, 231, 235, 242
mental illness, 140, 209
mercury toxicity, 250
miasms, 2–4, 33–34, 94–95
Michael (father), 52–54
migraines, 217
miscarriage, 140, 157
mistletoe, 92
morning sickness, 181
Mother Earth, 69, 99, 128, 139, 199
Mother Nature, 103
mother tinctures, 87
motherwort, 93, *190*, 191–93
mouth ulcers, 156
mucous, 160, 246
mugwort, 56, *194*, 195–97
mulberry bush, 72

mullein, *198*, 199–201
multiple sclerosis, 200
muscle apathy, 193
muscle relaxants, 153
muscle soreness, 208
muscle tension, 149

Native Americans, spirits in the Appalachians, 59–69
nausea, 152, 165, 226
near-death experiences, 34
negative spirits, 115, 163
nerve pain, 149, 164
nervous system, 133, 137, 213
nettles, 61–62, *202*, 203–5
Nin, Anaïs, 60
Nirvana, 101
non-judgement, 116, 212
nosebleeds, 140
nourishment, 98–99

offerings, 110–11
olive oil, 149
orphanage, 13
ovaries, 213
overwhelm, 199

pancreas, 173, 185, 250
paralysis, 238
parasites, 149, 188, 208, 218, 247
parasitic infection, 112–13
Parkinson's disease, 192
partnership, 116–17
patience, 167
peace, 132
personal growth, 69
pesticides, 10–11, 34, 87–92

petals, 100
petting zoo, 29
phlegm, 176
plague, 13
plant kingdom, 71
plants and plant spirits, 6–8, 15–16, 45–47, 73, 102–3. *See also specific plants*
  divine nature of, 98–106
  healing and, 103–6, 116–19
  journeying with, 107–11
  making plant spirit essences, 120–23
  physical properties of, 253–60
  spiritual and emotional properties, 260–67
plant spirit prayers. *See specific plants*
playful energy, 147
pneumonia, 184
poison ivy, 153
poison oak, 153
poke, 13–17, *206*, 207–9
pottery, 39
prayer, 12, 76, 107–8, 116–19, 121
pregnancy, 136, 140, 144, 230
pride, 151, 163
prostate, 132, 169
protection, 69, 131, 225
protection rituals, 26
psychic field, 131
pulsatilla, *210*, 211–13
purification, 114

queen bee, 175

rape, 75, 169
rashes, 152, 189, 200

reality, exploring, 116–17
reciprocity, law of, 103, 117
red chestnut, 72
red clover, *214*, 215–19
reincarnation, 12
remedies, 9
respect, 118
rest, 193
rites of passage, 21
ritualistic abuse, 33
rituals, 69
Robert (client), 47–57
rosemary, 36–37, *220*, 221–23
rue, 36–37, *224*, 225–27

sage, 39, *228*, 229–31
Sammie (stray cat), 88
scar tissue, 193
sciatica, 239
scorn, 203
Seattle (Chief), 25
sedatives, 234
seedlings, 98–99
seizures, 157, 168
self-absorption, 155, 204
self-compassion, 116
self-dignity, 151
self-forgiveness, 132
selflessness, 155
sepals, 99–100
sexual energy, 70, 148
sexually transmitted diseases, 219
sexual violence, 169
shaman, 5–9, 33, 39–40, 83–84, 96
shame, 216
shingles, 212
shock, 160

shut down, 136
sinus issues, 160, 172, 204, 216, 230, 234
skullcap, 53–54, *232*, 233–35
sleep, 239, 243
smoking, 217
Some, Malidoma, 17
sore throats, 223
soul, 16–17
soul loss, 136
souls, 33–34
spells, 131
Spirit, 99, 100–101, 105–6
spirit possession, 139
spleen, 173, 223, 250
spring water, 121
stems, 99
stimulants, 132
St. John's Wort, 44, 46–47, *236*, 237–39
stomach, 137, 188, 205
stress, 141
strokes, 168, 192
stuck souls, 31–32
supplements, 25

telepathy, 6
throat chakra, 233–34
throat infections, 164, 207–8
thymus gland, 145, 148
thyroid, 168, 239
tobacco, 79
tonsillitis, 235, 251
tooth pain, 153
torture, 75
toxins, 148
transitions, 183

trauma, 160
tribal dance, 76–77
tributes, 21
trust, 207–8
truth, 100, 250
tuberculosis, 14, 112–13, 209
tummy aches, 152
tumors, 141, 192–93

ulcers, 189, 193
unconscious, 116
urban shaman, 90
uterus, 132, 140–41, 149, 213, 227, 235, 239

varicose veins, 231
vibration, 103, 114
violet, 93, *240*, 241–43
viruses, 152
visions, 6
vitamin deficiencies, 136

vodka, 121
vomiting, 152

war, 180
warriors, 69, 75
water element, 108
Watson, Lyall, 29
weakness, 200
White Eagle, 116
womb, 98–99
women, 74–76
Wooden Leg, 68
worms, 135, 157, 188, 218
wormwood, *244*, 245–47
worry, 199
wounds, 189

yarrow, *248*, 249–52
yeast, 156, 172, 184, 185, 218, 247
yin/yang, 135

Books of Related Interest

Affirmations of the Light in Times of Darkness
Healing Messages from a Spiritwalker
by Laura Aversano

In this collection of inspired prayers and powerful affirmations, the author actively transmits her healing wisdom and spiritual support. Addressing trauma, depression, grief, anger, and revelation, her words awaken individual spiritual paths and provide solace and protection, leaving you forever transformed, initiated into the spiritual path of light, even in times of darkness.

Plant Spirit Healing
A Guide to Working with Plant Consciousness
by Pam Montgomery
Foreword by Stephen Harrod Buhner

Herbalist Pam Montgomery's triple spiral path—working through the heart to connect with the soul and gain access to the spirit—is a hands-on approach to partnering with plant spirits that promotes a profound healing, one that moves beyond mere symptomatic treatment into aligning us with the vast web of nature.

Communicating with Plants
Heart-Based Practices for Connecting with Plant Spirits
by Jen Frey
Foreword by Pam Montgomery

Everyone has an innate ability to consciously communicate with Plants. Jen Frey explains the synergistic process of communicating with Plants and how they can help us heal and teach us to trust, forgive, and embrace self-love. She also shares teachings from a variety of Plants such as Yarrow, Mugwort, Maple, Dandelion, and Poison Ivy.

Scan the QR code and save 25% at InnerTraditions.com. Browse over 2,000 titles on spirituality, the occult, ancient mysteries, new science, holistic health, and natural medicine.

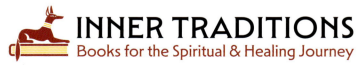

— SINCE 1975 • ROCHESTER, VERMONT —

InnerTraditions.com • (800) 246-8648